Contemporary Endocrinology

Series Editor

Leonid Poretsky
New York, NY, USA

Contemporary Endocrinology offers an array of titles covering clinical as well as bench research topics of interest to practicing endocrinologists and researchers. Topics include obesity management, androgen excess disorders, stem cells in endocrinology, evidence-based endocrinology, diabetes, genomics and endocrinology, as well as others. Series Editor Leonid Poretsky, MD, is Chief of the Division of Endocrinology and Associate Chairman for Research at Lenox Hill Hospital, and Professor of Medicine at Hofstra North Shore-LIJ School of Medicine.

More information about this series at http://www.springer.com/series/7680

William V. Tamborlane
Editor

Diabetes in Children and Adolescents

A Guide to Diagnosis and Management

Humana Press

Editor
William V. Tamborlane
Yale-New Haven Children's Hospital
Department of Pediatrics
Yale School of Medicine
New Haven, CT
USA

ISSN 2523-3785 ISSN 2523-3793 (electronic)
Contemporary Endocrinology
ISBN 978-3-030-64132-0 ISBN 978-3-030-64133-7 (eBook)
https://doi.org/10.1007/978-3-030-64133-7

This Humana imprint is published by the registered company Springer Nature Switzerland AG
The registered company address is: Gewerbestrasse 11, 6330 Cham, Switzerland

Special thanks to Susan Berson who has been a generous supporter of our Children's Diabetes Research Program for many years

Series Editor Foreword

Because type 1 diabetes afflicts a minority of patients with diabetes (approximately 10%), it is sometimes referred to as the "other type." Its importance, however, is impossible to overestimate, both because of its life-threatening nature and because it usually presents in childhood, therefore impacting immensely the affected person's entire life.

This book is devoted to diabetes mellitus in children. Although in Chap. 2 the authors discuss a variety of rare types of diabetes (mostly monogenetic in nature) that are seen in children, the majority of this volume focuses on type 1 and type 2 diabetes in childhood (type 2 diabetes has been seen with increasingly alarming frequency in children). The expert group of authors discusses in detail genetics, pathogenesis, clinical manifestations, therapeutic targets, and therapeutic tools available today for the management of diabetes mellitus in children.

This up-to-date book is highly recommended for pediatric endocrinologists who will, without doubt, find it invaluable in both their academic and clinical pursuits.

Leonid Poretsky
Division of Endocrinology
Lenox Hill Hospital
New York, NY, USA

Contents

Contributors

Sonia Caprio, MD Yale-New Haven Children's Hospital, Department of Pediatrics, Yale School of Medicine, New Haven, CT, USA

Lori Carria, SC Yale-New Haven Children's Hospital, Department of Pediatrics, Yale School of Medicine, New Haven, CT, USA

Eda Cengiz, MD, MHS Yale-New Haven Children's Hospital, Department of Pediatrics, Yale School of Medicine, New Haven, CT, USA

Ishani Choksi, MD Yale-New Haven Children's Hospital, Department of Pediatrics, Yale School of Medicine, New Haven, CT, USA

Elizabeth A. Doyle, DPN, APRN Yale School of Nursing, Primary Care Division, Orange, CT, USA

Patricia Gatcomb, MSN, APRN Yale-New Haven Children's Hospital, Department of Pediatrics, Yale School of Medicine, New Haven, CT, USA

Rachel Goldberg-Gel, MSN, CPNP, APRN Yale-New Haven Children's Hospital, Department of Pediatrics, Yale School of Medicine, New Haven, CT, USA

Cindy Guandalini, MSN Yale-New Haven Children's Hospital, Department of Pediatrics, Yale School of Medicine, New Haven, CT, USA

Jasmine Gujral, MD Yale-New Haven Children's Hospital, Department of Pediatrics, Yale School of Medicine, New Haven, CT, USA

Pamela Hu, MD Yale-New Haven Children's Hospital, Department of Pediatrics, Yale School of Medicine, New Haven, CT, USA

Kelly Joseph, MD Yale-New Haven Children's Hospital, Department of Pediatrics, Yale School of Medicine, New Haven, CT, USA

Patrick McAllister, BS University of Connecticut, School of Medicine, Farmington, CT, USA

Shana Mencher, MD Yale-New Haven Children's Hospital, Department of Pediatrics, Yale School of Medicine, New Haven, CT, USA

Kathryn Nagel, MD Yale New Haven Hospital, Internal Medicine/Pediatrics Residency, New Haven, CT, USA

Laura Nally, MD Yale-New Haven Children's Hospital, Department of Pediatrics, Yale School of Medicine, New Haven, CT, USA

Amy Page, LCSW Yale Children's Hospital, Social Work, New Haven, CT, USA

Anisha Patel, DO Yale-New Haven Children's Hospital, Department of Pediatrics, Yale School of Medicine, New Haven, CT, USA

Rachel Perry, MD Yale University School of Medicine, Cellular & Molecular Physiology and Internal Medicine (Endocrinology), New Haven, CT, USA

Paulina Rose, RD, CDCES Yale-New Haven Children's Hospital, Department of Pediatrics, Yale School of Medicine, New Haven, CT, USA

Stephanie Samuels, MD Yale-New Haven Children's Hospital, Department of Pediatrics, Yale School of Medicine, New Haven, CT, USA

Nicola Santoro, MD Yale-New Haven Children's Hospital, Department of Pediatrics, Yale School of Medicine, New Haven, CT, USA

Mary Savoye, RD, CDCES Yale-New Haven Children's Hospital, Department of Pediatrics, Yale School of Medicine, New Haven, CT, USA

Jennifer Sherr, MD Yale-New Haven Children's Hospital, Department of Pediatrics, Yale School of Medicine, New Haven, CT, USA

Stephan Siebel, MD Yale-New Haven Children's Hospital, Department of Pediatrics, Yale School of Medicine, New Haven, CT, USA

Amy Steffen, BSN, RN Yale-New Haven Children's Hospital, Department of Pediatrics, Yale School of Medicine, New Haven, CT, USA

Kerry Stephenson, MSN Yale-New Haven Children's Hospital, Department of Pediatrics, Yale School of Medicine, New Haven, CT, USA

William V. Tamborlane, MD Yale-New Haven Children's Hospital, Department of Pediatrics, Yale School of Medicine, New Haven, CT, USA

Eileen Tichy, RD, PA Yale-New Haven Children's Hospital, Department of Pediatrics, Yale School of Medicine, New Haven, CT, USA

Michelle Van Name, MD Yale-New Haven Children's Hospital, Department of Pediatrics, Yale School of Medicine, New Haven, CT, USA

Apoorva Ravindranath Waikar, MD Yale-New Haven Children's Hospital, Department of Pediatrics, Yale School of Medicine, New Haven, CT, USA

Stuart A. Weinzimer, MD Yale-New Haven Children's Hospital, Department of Pediatrics, Yale School of Medicine, New Haven, CT, USA

Melinda Zgorski, BSN Yale-New Haven Children's Hospital, Department of Pediatrics, Yale School of Medicine, New Haven, CT, USA

Part I

Type 1 Diabetes

Introduction

1

William V. Tamborlane

Introduction

To paraphrase Charles Dickens, it has been the best of times, as well as the worst of times, for youth with type 1 diabetes (T1D). As will be described in the first section of this book, there has been a virtual explosion in the development of advanced diabetes technologies during the past 20 years, such as new and improved insulin pumps and more accurate, real-time continuous glucose monitors (CGMs) for youth with T1D. Indeed, CGMs have been approved for use as a replacement for blood glucose meter measurements and begun to fill the full potential of insulin pump therapy by its incorporation into semi-automatic integrated insulin pump/glucose sensor systems. In these systems, insulin pump infusion rates are partially regulated automatically by changes in sensor glucose concentrations transmitted to mini-computers imbedded in the patient's insulin pump. The first integrated devices that have been approved by regulatory agencies have been called *hybrid closed-loop systems* because patients still must activate their pumps manually to administer large boluses of insulin

W. V. Tamborlane (✉)
Yale-New Haven Children's Hospital, Department of Pediatrics,
Yale School of Medicine, New Haven, CT, USA
e-mail: William.tamborlane@yale.edu

W. V. Tamborlane (ed.), *Diabetes in Children and Adolescents*, Contemporary Endocrinology,
https://doi.org/10.1007/978-3-030-64133-7_1

prior to meals and large snacks. However, changes in the rate of insulin infusion between meals and during the overnight period are controlled automatically based on changes in sensor glucose readings. *There no longer are pre-programed basal infusion rates when these systems are running under automatic control between meals and during the overnight period.* Moreover, integrated and stand-alone CGMs can transmit sensor data to the cloud and have those data transmitted to smart phones. Such devices are very popular with parents of young children with type 1 diabetes because they can follow changes in their child's glucose levels over their phones in real time.

Nevertheless, too many youth with T1D fail to make use of new advanced diabetes technologies, HbA1c levels remain too high, and episodes of severe hypoglycemia and diabetes ketoacidosis occur too often, especially in adolescents with T1D.

Additionally, a plethora of drugs in more than four new drug classes have been approved for use in adults with type 2 diabetes (T2D). Until recently, however, the only drug that was approved for use in children and adolescents with T2D that was based on the results of a small randomized clinical trial was metformin, a drug that was approved for use in youth with T2D more than 20 years ago. In the second section of this book, we will explain why it has been so difficult to successfully complete randomized clinical trials to demonstrate the efficacy and safety of new drugs in youth with T2D. We will also indicate that we may be about to transform the treatment of pediatric T2D in the near future.

Putting Advances in Treatment of T1D in Perspective

At the successful completion of the Diabetes Control and Complications Trial (DCCT), which demonstrated the ability of intensive therapy to delay or prevent the development of diabetes complications in 1993, the DCCT Chair, Oscar Crofford, said, "This is not the beginning of the end of T1D but rather the end of the beginning of trying to effectively manage T1D." Dr. Crofford foresaw the many challenges that patients and practitioners still faced in achieving and maintaining improved outcomes of diabetes. With this in mind, it is worthwhile to briefly review how far we have advanced in treating youth with T1D.

I began my postdoctoral fellowship in pediatric endocrinology at Yale in 1975, having just completed pediatric residency at Georgetown University. As chief resident at Georgetown, I helped institute a new way to treat children and adolescents with T1D who were admitted to the hospital for treatment of diabetic ketoacidosis. The new method of low-dose intravenous infusions of regular insulin (instead of large subcutaneous injections of insulin) was based on a paper by Professor George Alberti and colleagues published in the *British Medical Journal* [1]. Consequently, this approach has become the well-established standard of care for treatment of diabetic ketoacidosis. As a result, treatment of diabetes became an area of special interest for me [2].

Unfortunately, I didn't realize how poor the treatment of youth withT1D was at that time. Specifically, regular, NPH, and Lente were the only insulins available and these were injected only once or twice a day. These agents were produced from insulin that was extracted from beef and pork pancreases, and their time-action profiles did not match the rates of carbohydrate absorption during meals and they were full of impurities that contributed to the development of lipoatrophy at injection sites. Even the syringes being used during in the 1960s and 1970s pale in comparison to today's pens and tiny microneedles.

In what I like to call the "Bad Old Days of Diabetes," we also did not have an effective way of monitoring treatment, since self-blood glucose meter monitoring wasn't invented until 1979–1980. Instead, for years, youngsters were instructed to check the presence or absence of glucose in their urine, three or four times a day. In retrospect, this was a totally worthless endeavor. According to one of our parents, "adjusting insulin doses based on monitoring urine glucose is like trying to hit a baseball by its shadow." Another parent told me, "it's like driving a car that only registers speeds over 180 miles/hour." One of the early pioneers in the development of blood glucose monitoring had T1D, himself. He told me that he started measuring fingerstick blood glucose levels because he couldn't understand why he felt like he was hypoglycemic even when his urine still tested positive for glucose.

Of course, we tortured our T1D patients even further by asking them to collect all of their urine on the day prior to their scheduled visit, in four separate aliquots: breakfast to lunch, lunch to dinner, dinner to bedtime, and overnight. We even scheduled our diabetes clinics on Monday, so families could bring in these collections immediately after the weekend. Incredibly, we often adjusted breakfast and dinner insulin doses based on 1 day of urine collections—ALSO WORTHLESS! In retrospect, in those days, we simply gave enough insulin to encourage normal growth and to prevent diabetic ketoacidosis. It's no surprise that once we were able to measure HbA1c levels, almost all of our patients had values that were >11.0%.

Turning the Corner

1979–1980 saw the introduction of the first tools that provided more physiologic insulin delivery and better ways to monitor blood glucose control. Our contribution was to show that the continuous subcutaneous infusion of insulin by a miniaturized infusion pump was a more physiologic and effective method of replacement of insulin in T1D than one or two daily injections of insulin [3]. The success of insulin pump therapy was followed by the introduction of multiple daily injections of short- and long-acting insulins; both pumps and injections came to be known as basal/bolus therapy. At the same time, the ability to monitor the effectiveness of treatment of diabetes was transformed by the introduction of self-monitoring of blood glucose (SMBG) and the realization that measuring glycosylated hemoglobin (especially HbA1c) provided a simple test that reflected average blood glucose levels over the past 3 months.

These advances made the DCCT possible, since we were able to achieve and maintain HbA1c levels that were substantially lower in participants randomized to the intensive treatment group than the conventional treatment group during the 10 years of that study (Fig. 1.1). Even more important, the DCCT conclusively established

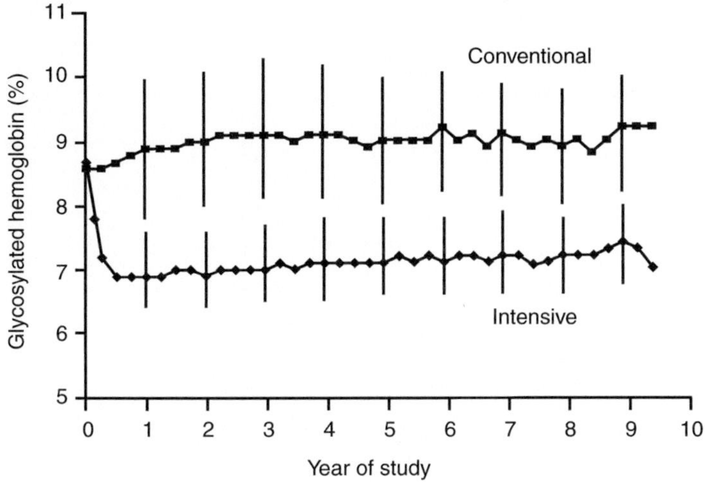

Fig. 1.1 Differences in HbA1c levels in patients randomized to the conventional and intensive treatment groups in the 10 years of treatment in the Diabetes Control and Complications Trial (DCCT). (From the DCCT Study Group (Ref. [4] below))

that lowering blood glucose and HbA1c to levels as close to normal as possible could delay or prevent the development of diabetic retinopathy (the primary outcome of that study), as well as other diabetes-related vascular complications [4, 5]. Long-term follow-up of DCCT participants in the Epidemiology of Diabetes Interventions and Complications (EDIC) study has continued to demonstrate the benefits of strict metabolic control [6, 7]. One of the truly amazing aspects of DCCT/EDIC is that nearly all participants have continued to be seen for follow-up for more than 35 years.

So, What's the Problem?

While most of the participants who were randomized to the intensive treatment group in the DCCT did very well in achieving strict metabolic control of diabetes. The rate of severe hypoglycemia increased by threefold, especially in individuals with the lowest HbA1c levels [4]. Moreover, the assistance and encouragement

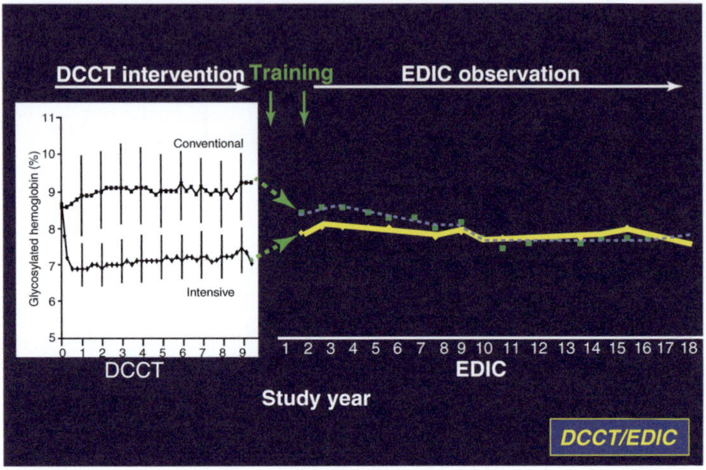

Fig. 1.2 Changes in HbA1c in the two former treatment groups in EDIC

provided to participants by our dedicated cadre of nurse coordinators played a very important role in the success of the DCCT, which was difficult to simulate in clinical practice. Indeed, HbA1c levels increased from ~7.0 to ~8.0% in the prior intensive treatment group when they returned to regular clinical practice, whereas HbA1c fell from ~9.0 to only 8.0% in the former conventional group who received training in intensive treatment at the end of the DCCT (Fig. 1.2).

Consequently, considerable effort has been spent over the past 27 years to increase the efficacy of insulin treatment without increasing the rates of severe hypoglycemia. These efforts have resulted in the introduction of both fast-acting and long-acting insulin analogs, increased use of new and improved insulin pumps, and development of real-time continuous glucose monitors of sufficient accuracy to replace the need for SMBG testing. It should be noted, however, that none of these advances reduced the burdens of managing T1D or parental fears of hypoglycemia and diabetic ketoacidosis.

The continuing challenges of treatment of T1D, especially in adolescents, is well illustrated by initial data collected regarding clinical outcomes in the T1D Exchange Clinic Registry of >26,000 patients with T1D in the USA [8]. Across all age groups, teenagers between 13 and 18 years of age had the highest HbA1c levels, reaching values just below 9.0%, not far removed from baseline HbA1c levels of teenagers enrolled in the DCCT more than 35 years ago. Indeed, few patients in this age group achieved target HbA1c levels <7.5% and it took until age 30 for HbA1c levels to fall to values seen in older adults (i.e., ~7.5%). I like to call this the *"Peter Pan"* scenario, namely, young adult males who fail to mature until past 30 years of age. Moreover, follow-up data from the T1D Exchange Registry showed that HbA1c levels actually increased in adolescents, the risk of severe hypoglycemia and DKA remained high, and ≤50% of pediatric patients were using advanced diabetes technologies [9].

Is There a Light at the End of the Tunnel?

My colleagues and I strongly believe that we are poised at the edge of transformational advances in the treatment of youth with T1D, namely, significant advances in therapy that improve clinical outcomes, while simultaneously decreasing the burdens of diabetes treatment. Consequently, we have dedicated the first section of this book to a number of chapters describing the advances that have had the greatest impact on the treatment of youth with T1D, including the state of the art in insulin pumps, the newest generation of continuous glucose monitoring (CGM) devices, and, most importantly, the integration of CGM into semi-automatic, hybrid insulin pump/CGM systems.

Our book chapters will cover bread and butter issues like the following:

- The pathophysiology of type 1 and type 2 diabetes
- Diagnosing diabetes
- Initial management of youth with type 1 diabetes
- Types and actions of different insulins
- Insulin pump therapy
- Monitoring glycemic control

Important educational and life-style factors like the following:

- Medical nutrition therapy
- Exercise and diabetes
- Psychosocial challenges of T1D

Other factors like the following:

- Acute complications of diabetes
- Sick day management
- Screening for co-morbidities
- Adjunctive therapies not named insulin
- Screening for co-morbidities
- Patients' views of the challenges of managing T1D as a child and adolescent
- Automated insulin delivery systems

What About Pediatric Type 2 Diabetes (T2D)?

The obesity epidemic in the USA and around the world has been accompanied by the relatively recent discovery that obese youngsters can develop T2D, usually between the age of 10 and 18 years. Consequently, we have committed the second section of this book to the challenges of caring for youth with T2D. The TODAY study demonstrated that most adolescents with new-onset T2D can be adequately managed by metformin alone, even if they require initial treatment with insulin to rapidly correct glucotoxicity [10]. However, the TODAY study also demonstrated that metformin monotherapy often fails rapidly, requiring addition of a second drug to maintain target HbA1c levels [11]. While adults with T2D have a plethora of choices of new drugs for add-on treatment to metformin, insulin was the only other drug approved for use in youth with T2D for the past 20 years. Unfortunately, the efficacy of insulin for rescue treatment of youth with T2D has generally been disappointing for many reasons. Consequently, it is very encouraging that treatment choices for youth with T2D are beginning to expand, as illustrated by the approval of use of the GLP1 agonist, liraglutide [12], and the approaching completion of several other pivotal trials of other new drugs for treatment of youth with T2D [13]. Since virtually all youth with T2D are obese or overweight, the approval of new medications for treatment of obesity may also benefit youth with T2D. Hopefully, we're about to turn the corner from the worst to the best decade for treatment of pediatric T2D; only time will tell.

References

1. Page MM, Alberti KG, Greenword R, Gumaa KA, Lowy C, Nabarro JD, Pyke DA, Sonksen PH, Watkins PJ, West TE. Treatment of diabetic coma with continuous low-dose infusion of insulin. Br Med J. 1974;2:687–90.
2. Tamborlane WV, Genel M. Discordant correction of hyperglycemia and ketoacidosis with low-dose insulin infusion. Pediatrics. 1978;61:125–7.
3. Tamborlane WV, Sherwin RS, Genel M, Felig P. Reduction to normal of plasma glucose in juvenile diabetics by subcutaneous administration of insulin with a portable infusion pump. N Engl J Med. 1979;300:573–8.
4. The DCCT Research Group. The effect of intensive diabetes treatment on the development and progression of long-term complications in insulin-dependent diabetes mellitus. The Diabetes Control and Complications Trial. N Engl J Med. 1993;329:977–86.
5. The DCCT Research Group. The effect of intensive diabetes treatment on the development and progression of long-term complications in adolescents with insulin-dependent diabetes mellitus: the Diabetes Control and Complications Trial. J Pediatr. 1994;125:177–88.
6. Nathan DM. for the DCCT/EDIC Research Group. The diabetes control and complications trial/epidemiology of diabetes interventions and complications study at 30 years: overview. Diabetes Care. 2014;37:9–16.
7. DCCT/EDIC Research Group. Retinopathy and nephropathy in patients with type 1 diabetes four years after a trial of intensive therapy. N Engl J Med. 2000;342:381–9.
8. Miller KM, Foster NC, Beck RW, Bergenstal RM, Dubose S, DiMeglio LA, Maahs DM, Tamborlane WV. Current state of type 1 diabetes treatment in the US: updated data from the T1D exchange clinic registry. Diabetes Care. 2015;38:971–8.
9. Foster NC, Miller KM, DiMeglio LA, Maahs DM, Tamborlane WV, Bergenstal R, Clements M, Rickels MR, Smith E, Olson BA, Garg SK, Beck RW. State of type 1 diabetes management and outcomes from the T1D exchange in 2016-2018: comparison with 2010-2012. Diabetes Technol Ther. 2019;21:66–72.

10. Laffel L, Chang N, Grey M, Hale D, Higgins L, Hirst K, Izquierdo R, Larkin M, Macha C, Pham T, Wauters A, Weinstock RS. for the TODAY Study Group. Metformin monotherapy in youth with recent onset type 2 diabetes: experience from the prerandomization run-in phase of the TODAY study. Pediatr Diabetes. 2012;13:369–73.
11. TODAY Study Group, Zeitler P, Hirst K, Pyle L, Linder B, Copeland K, Arslanian S, Cuttler L, Nathan DM, Tollefsen S, Wilfley D, Kaufman F. A clinical trial to maintain glycemic control in youth with type 2 diabetes. N Engl J Med. 2012;366:2247–56.
12. Tamborlane WV, Fainberg U, Frimer-Larsen H, Hafez M, Hale PM, Jalaludin MY, Kovarenko M, Libman I, Lynch J, Rao PV, Shehadeh N, Turan S, Weghuber D, Barrientos-Pérez M, Barrett T. Liraglutide in children and adolescents with type 2 diabetes. NEJM. 2019;381:637–46.
13. Van Name M, Klingensmith K, Nelson B, Wintergerst K, Mitchell J, Norris K. Tamborlane WV for the Pediatric Diabetes Consortium. Transforming performance of clinical trials in pediatric type 2 diabetes – a consortium model. Diabetes technology and therapeutics. Diabetes Technol Ther. 2020;22:330–6.

Pathophysiology of Types of Pediatric and Adolescent Diabetes

2

Stephan Siebel, Pamela Hu, and Rachel Perry

Introduction

Diabetes mellitus encompasses a group of multifactorial, genetically heterogeneous metabolic disorders all of which result in defective glucose metabolism secondary to absolute or relative insulinopenia or both. Even though the etiology may vary among different types of diabetes, they all share a common pathophysiology of hyperglycemia, leading to polyuria, polydipsia, weight loss, and eventually resulting in microvascular and macrovascular complications that increase morbidity and mortality for people with diabetes. Table 2.1 summarizes the different types of diabetes.

S. Siebel (✉) · P. Hu
Yale-New Haven Children's Hospital, Department of Pediatrics, Yale School of Medicine, New Haven, CT, USA
e-mail: Stephan.siebel@yale.edu; pamela.hu@yale.edu

R. Perry
Yale University School of Medicine, Cellular & Molecular Physiology and Internal Medicine (Endocrinology), New Haven, CT, USA
e-mail: rachel.perry@yale.edu

W. V. Tamborlane (ed.), *Diabetes in Children and Adolescents*, Contemporary Endocrinology,
https://doi.org/10.1007/978-3-030-64133-7_2

Table 2.1 Different type of diabetes

Types of diabetes	Description
Type 1 diabetes (T1D)	There are two forms of type 1 diabetes: 1a (immune-mediated) and 1b (idiopathic). The etiology, pathogenesis, and pathophysiology will be discussed in this chapter
Type 2 diabetes (T2D)	Most common form of diabetes in adults characterized by hyperglycemia and insulin resistance whose prevalence increases with degrees of obesity. T2DM will be further discussed in this chapter
Monogenic forms of diabetes	
Neonatal diabetes	Transient or permanent monogenic form of diabetes that occurs in newborns through first 6 months of life. Incidence of 1 in 100,000–500,000 live births. Multiple genes are known to be affected. Treatment may be insulin or sulfonylureas and some conditions may affect pancreatic exocrine function as well
Monogenic diabetes of the young (MODY)	Heterogeneous group of dominantly inherited noninsulin-dependent diabetes diagnosed at age <25 years. Patients do not have autoantibodies and have one of many identified genetic abnormalities that affect the development, function, and regulation of beta cells. Most common monogenic form of diabetes, 2–5% prevalence Most common: HNF1A mutation in 52–65% MODY cases, glucokinase gene mutation in 15–32% MODY cases
Mitochondrial diabetes	Rare mitochondrial disorder that causes insulin-dependent diabetes and deafness. The most common and best described mtDNA mutation which encodes tRNA is A3243G that results in defect in insulin secretion. Age of onset is 30–40 years and onset of diabetes is usually preceded by development of bilateral sensorineural hearing and retinitis pigmentosa
Genetic defects in insulin action	Rare disorders such as leprechaunism, type A insulin resistance, Rabson-Mendenhall (RM) syndrome, and Donahue syndrome cause severe insulin resistance. The latter three disorders are due to defects in the *INSR* gene that encodes the insulin receptor. Type A is the milder and more common of the three (1 in 100,000), whereas RM syndrome and Donahue syndrome occur in less than one per million.

Table 2.1 (continued)

Types of diabetes	Description
Cystic fibrosis–related diabetes (CFRD)	Common complication of cystic fibrosis is due to pancreatic exocrine deficiency. Recommended screening for diabetes starts at age 10 years. Primary cause is insulin deficiency is due to destruction of pancreatic islets in addition to insulin resistance in setting of repeated acute exacerbations or worsening lung function
Drug- or chemical-induced diabetes	Many medications affect glucose tolerance. They can decrease insulin secretion, increase hepatic gluconeogenesis, or cause insulin resistance. These include, but are not limited to, first- and second-generation anti-psychotics, anti-infectives including fluoroquinolones and HIV antiretrovirals, many cardiovascular drugs such as beta blockers, thiazides, diazoxide, epinephrine, glucocorticoids, immunosuppressants
Genetic syndromes associated with diabetes – there are many genetic conditions associated with diabetes, and only a few are described below:	
Wolfram syndrome	Also known as DIDMOAD (diabetes insipidus, diabetes mellitus, optic atrophy, deafness). Autosomal recessive inheritance of mutated WSF1. 1 in 150 patients with type 1 diabetes
Lipodystrophic diabetes	Clinically diverse group of disorders characterized by complete or partial lack of adipose tissue associated with severe insulin resistance possibly due to absence or defects of insulin receptor expression, function, or signaling
X-linked polyendocrinopathy, immune dysfunction and diarrhea (XPID)	In this rare x-linked recessive condition, lymphocytes invade multiple organs including the pancreas resulting in insulitis and beta-cell destruction. Mutation in the *FOXP3* gene results in lack of regulatory T cells and overwhelming autoimmunity. When diagnosed early, child may receive therapeutic benefit from bone marrow transplantation to restore functional T-regulatory cells

Normal Physiology of the β-Cell's Secretion of Insulin

The endocrine pancreas is made up of islets of Langerhans which contribute up to 3% of the total pancreatic volume. There are ~3 million islet cells, of which 60% are insulin producing β-cells. When glucose enters the β-cell through insulin-independent GLUT 2 transporters, it is phosphorylated by glucokinase and subsequently metabolized to produce ATP via glycolysis and cellular respiration. Phosphorylation by glucokinase is a rate-limiting step of glycolysis, and defects affecting this enzyme can decrease the glucose sensitivity of a β-cells. The increasing ATP/ADP ratio within β-cells closes the ATP sensitive potassium channel. Closure of the potassium channels results in intracellular accumulation of potassium and depolarization of β-cells. This in turn leads to opening of voltage-gated Ca^{2+} channels Cav 1.2/1.3. Influx of Ca^{2+} promotes fusion of insulin granules with the plasma membrane resulting in exocytosis of insulin.

Insulin, a peptide hormone, is one of the key regulators of glucose homeostasis. It is synthesized as pre-proinsulin, which is then converted into proinsulin. Proinsulin consists of an α and a β-chain, which are connected together by C-peptide. During posttranslational modifications, proinsulin is cleaved by carboxypeptidase into insulin and c-peptide, which are stored within insulin granules and co-secreted into the systemic circulation upon β-cell depolarization. Maturation of proinsulin to insulin through the cleavage of C-peptide only occurs in the pancreatic β-cells. Up to 3% of intact proinsulin can be secreted into the systemic circulation, whereas C-peptide is secreted in nearly equimolar ratios with endogenous insulin.

Insulin secretion and sensitivity vary throughout a 24-hour period. Hyperglycemic clamp studies and IV glucose tolerance tests have shown that insulin is secreted in two distinct phases from the beta cell. During the "rapid" first phase, preformed insulin granules are secreted within 3–5 min of β-cell depolarization. If glucose exposure continues beyond this first phase, further insulin is released from stored and newly synthesized insulin granules. This "sustained" second phase of insulin secretion is mediated by Cav 2.3. Impaired first phase has been determined to

Table 2.2 Insulin-mediated glucose clearance

Target tissue	Insulin action
Muscle	Increases glucose uptake and metabolism via translocation of GLUT4 from an intracellular pool to the surface of the cells Promotes protein synthesis by the uptake of amino acids and suppresses atrophy
Adipose	Increases glucose uptake Increases lipogenesis through uptake of triglycerides and suppresses lipolysis
Liver	Promotes lipogenesis through uptake of triglycerides Counters action of glucagon which then suppresses gluconeogenesis

be a very sensitive marker of early beta-cell dysfunction and is seen as predictive of diabetes onset [1].

Once secreted, insulin interacts with membrane-bound tyrosine kinase cell-surface receptors which are located throughout the body. Insulin receptors consist of four subunits (two alpha-subunits and two beta-subunits) and are similar in structure to the IGF-1 receptor. Once insulin binds the alpha-subunits, the intracellular tyrosine kinase domains of the beta-subunits are activated and phosphorylate intracellular partners of specific tyrosine residues. Once the receptor is phosphorylated, adaptor proteins, such as insulin receptor substrates (IRSs), interact with the receptor to propagate downstream signaling. This ultimately modulates cellular metabolism and stimulates mitogenesis and receptor internalization (Table 2.2).

In addition to its classical actions, insulin has an important effect on neuronal tissue, endothelial cells, cardiomyocytes, and immune cells such as macrophages. However, these roles are beyond the scope of this chapter.

β-Cell Dysfunction and Reduced Mass as Basis for Hyperglycemia Associated with Diabetes

In general, in diabetes mellitus, β-cell function and mass deteriorate over time leading to impaired glucose sensitivity and decreased insulin secretion, as well as overall disruption of β-cell architecture and structural integrity, all of which eventually result in hyperglycemia.

Type 1 Diabetes

Type 1 diabetes is divided into type 1a (autoimmune) and type 1b (idiopathic). Here we focus on type 1a. In type 1a diabetes (T1D), chronic autoimmune destruction of pancreatic β-cells is the primary pathologic process that results in insulinopenia and eventually in chronic hyperglycemia. Insulitis, or a peri-islet cellular infiltrate seen microscopically, was first described in the early nineteenth century and has been associated with reduction in β-cell mass and function. Four anti-islet autoantibodies have been described as highly sensitive markers for the diagnosis of T1D: anti-insulin, anti-glutamic acid decarboxylase, anti-insulinoma-associated antigen 2, and anti-zinc transporter 8 antibodies.

The presence of islet cell autoantibodies begins years before disease onset and overt metabolic decompensation. More than ninety percent of Caucasian children with T1D have at least one positive islet cell autoantibody. Two or more positive antibodies are pathognomic for development of T1D [2]. In addition to the presence of islet-cell antibodies, many genetic and environmental factors are known and hypothesized to impact a person's likelihood of developing T1D.

To date, the strongest predictive factors for diabetes have been linked to human leukocyte antigen (HLA), a group of cell surface proteins that mediate immune responses. These antigens are encoded by genes of the major histocompatibility complex (MHC). Allelic variation of these genes is associated with either susceptibility for or protection against developing diabetes. The most important loci determining T1D risk are located within the MHC on chromosome 6p21, particularly HLA class II molecules (DR, DQ, DP). Approximately 1 of 16 children with the highest-risk HLA genotype progresses to T1D as compared to a population risk of 1 per 300. Genetic factors also influence the expression of anti-islet autoantibodies.

T1D is a highly heterogeneous disease entity as shown by studies of monozygotic twins. Despite sharing the same genotype, overall concordance rates for T1D in identical twins are less 100% and vary depending on age of onset. For example, the concordance rate is higher in monozygotic twins when one twin develops diabetes at a younger age (<5 years) and lower when the index twin develops diabetes at an age greater than 25 years. This suggests that both environmental factors and non-germline-inherited variations contribute to the lifetime risk of developing diabetes.

Stages of Development of T1D Prior to T1D disease onset, there is a well-studied natural history of pre-T1D which has been described as two stages prior to disease onset. In stage 1, an individual has two or more anti-islet autoantibodies with normoglycemia. In stage 2, there is impaired glucose tolerance with two or more anti-islet autoantibodies. In stage 3, a patient meets ADA criteria for the diagnosis of diabetes.

Environmental Factors While genetic and autoimmune factors determine one's risk of developing T1DM, environmental factors also play an important role in the development of diabetes. Monozygotic twins have discordant rates of disease and onset can be temporally divergent. It is known that local disease rates assimilate when individuals migrate from low- to high-incidence countries. These facts, along with increasing rates of T1D worldwide, indicate environmental influences that factor into disease onset.

Viral infections are hypothesized to play a role in triggering autoimmunity that can subsequently lead to β-cell destruction and T1DM. Animal studies have shown possible mechanistic ways in which immune responses to viruses, particularly enteroviruses, may lead to autoimmunity against β-cells. Four mechanisms have been proposed: perturbation of thymic T-cell education, β-cell specific infection, bystander activation, and molecular mimicry [3]. Molecular mimicry, a mechanism whereby epitopes shared between viruses and β-cells result in cross-reactive immunity, has gained the most traction. It is thought to be unlikely to cause autoimmune diabetes in an otherwise unaffected person but rather trigger and accelerate disease progression in an otherwise predisposed individual.

Other environmental factors including diet, endocrine disruptors, and gut microbiome composition are also associated with T1D, as well as T2D. Dietary factors such as cow's milk and early exposure to cereals have been implicated in increasing risk of T1D, while exposure to cod liver oil and vitamin D supplements may be protective [4, 5]. Obesity and insulin resistance may factor not only into T2D but also the onset of T1D. Perinatal risk factors, vitamin D deficiency, and environmental polluters have also been implicated in the onset of T1D. Further research is needed to identify how these and other environmental factors play a role in disease development.

Type 2 Diabetes

Type 2 diabetes (T2D) is a multifactorial metabolic disorder with a strong genetic component, as exemplified by the high concordance rate among identical twins and a much stronger family history of T2D in affected individuals. It has been reported that anywhere from 74% to 100% of patients with T2D have a first- or second-degree relative with the disease, compared to 5% of patients with T1D. In T2D, peripheral insulin resistance leads to the inability of pancreatic β-cells to meet the increasing insulin requirements resulting in relative and eventually to absolute insulinopenia. The development of insulin resistance and β-cell dysfunction is a complex interaction between genetic and environmental factors that is still under investigation.

Many genes have been associated with T2D but their exact role in disease development remains to be clarified. Likewise, many environmental factors are closely associated with T2D development, namely excess caloric intake, obesity, as well as factors such as sleep disruption, stress, microbiome changes, and medications. There are also suspected epigenetic markers that can occur in early life that increase the risk of T2D development later in life. While specific genes have not clearly been defined as causative, there appears to be genetic influences on the development of T2D. The lifetime risk for a first-degree relative of a patient with

T2D is 5 to 10 times higher than that of age- and weight-matched subjects without a family history of diabetes. First-degree relatives of patients with T2D frequently have impaired non-oxidative glucose metabolism, indicative of insulin resistance, long before they develop T2D. In addition, they may have β-cell dysfunction, as evidenced by decreases in insulin and amylin release in response to glucose stimulation.

Ultimately insulin resistance plays a central role in the development of T2D. Insulin resistance refers to when insulin secretion does not have the same biologic effect as in a normal physiologic state. As reviewed earlier, insulin acts in myriad ways in muscle, fat, and hepatic tissue to maintain glucose homeostasis as well as protein and lipid homeostasis. Insulin resistance thus manifests as decreased glucose uptake and metabolism in muscle, impaired insulin suppression of lipolysis, and impaired ability to suppress hepatic gluconeogenesis.

Genetic Factors To date, genome-wide association studies have identified more than 100 susceptibility genes. However, these genetic variants explain less than 15% disease heritability; one example of a gene variant known to increase disease susceptibility is transcription factor gene TCF7L2. TCF7L2 variants increased the risk of progression from impaired glucose tolerance to T2D. The population-attributable risk for diabetes for this gene is estimated at 21 percent. That said, the polymorphism most associated with diabetes is an intronic variant and how or whether this affects expression of TCF7L2 mRNA or protein remains unknown.

Two other loci (rs7903146 and rs12255372) have been found to increase the risk of T2D in multiple populations in Iceland, Denmark, and the United States. Compared to non-carriers, carriers of the at-risk alleles had a relative risk for type 2 diabetes – 1.45 for heterozygotes and 2.41 for homozygotes.

Environmental Factors Many environmental factors are associated with T2D including excessive caloric intake leading to obesity, circadian rhythm disruption, inflammation, changes to the microbiome, and medications.

Pathophysiology of Hyperglycemia and Ketogenesis

In all known forms of diabetes, carbohydrate, protein, and lipid metabolisms are altered due to absolute or relative insulinopenia. The resultant hyperglycemia, proteolysis, and lipid oxidation/ketogenesis lead to acute and long-term complications. The immediate pathophysiology is caused by hyperglycemia due to impaired glucose uptake in the liver, adipose, and muscle cells and increased glycogenolysis and gluconeogenesis. When the serum glucose concentration exceeds the renal threshold for glucose (180 mg/dl or 10 mmol/L), glycosuria occurs. This osmotic diuresis leads to polyuria, promoting renal electrolyte loss and hypovolemia. The increasing serum osmolarity is sensed by hypothalamic osmoreceptors resulting in polydipsia.

With ongoing insulinopenia, alteration of carbohydrate, protein, and lipid metabolisms results in significant weight loss secondary to loss of water and calories with glycosuria along with whole body catabolism, manifested by breakdown of fat and muscle tissues.

Due to its strong inhibitory effect on hormone-sensitive lipase and beta oxidation, insulin deficiency leads to an increase of lipolysis followed by a rise in plasma free fatty acid ketone bodies.

Due to their high acidity, ketone bodies quickly use up the body's alkali reserve leading to metabolic acidosis. This is compensated for by respiratory mechanisms known as Kussmaul breathing. This deep, labored breathing pattern is a type of hyperventilation by which the body exhales CO_2 trying to balance the pH. As the physiologic stress continues, endogenous secretion of stress hormones (glucagon, catecholamines, cortisol, growth hormone) further increases lipolysis, proteolysis, glycogenolysis, and gluconeogenesis.

This severe state of ketotic, acidotic hyperglycemia is diabetic ketoacidosis (DKA), which has been defined in new onset patients as a blood glucose level >200 mg/dL (>11.1 mmol/L), venous pH less than 7.3 or serum bicarbonate level less than 15 mEq/L (<15 mmol/L), ketonemia (blood β-hydroxybutyrate concentration ≥3 mmol/L), and ketonuria. With evolving ketoacidosis, patients typically present with fruity-smelling breath due to acetone, nausea, vomiting, functional ileus, headaches, blurry vision, and lethargy. DKA can result in altered mental status/coma, cerebral edema, and death if not treated carefully and promptly.

In a newly diagnosed pediatric patient, classic symptoms of polyuria and polydipsia are present in more than 90% of patients, while the more severe presentation of diabetic ketoacidosis occurs in approximately 25–30% of newly diagnosed patients [6].

Over time, particularly in chronic states of hyperglycemia, small vessel disease occurs because glucose can enter vascular and nerve tissues without the assistance of insulin. This results in retinopathy, nephropathy, and neuropathy. Thus, glucose levels in these tissues will be as high as the plasma levels. The damage occurs because of the processes by which these tissues try to clear the glucose. Namely, three mechanisms: polyol pathway, enzymatic glycosylation and non-enzymatic glycosylation, result in vascular and neural tissue damage.

In a healthy state, glucose will be taken up by a cell, undergo glycolysis, and produce energy in the form of ATP through the Krebs cycle. In an insulin-deficient state, glucose will be taken up by a cell and will undergo enzymatic glycosylation. This converts glucose into glucose-1-phosphate which is transferred to proteins of the basement membrane and weakens the membrane leading to leakage of proteins, e.g., proteinuria seen in diabetic nephropathy, fluorescein leak seen in diabetic retinopathy, and albumin leak seen in peripheral artery disease.

The polyol pathway is another alternate glucose metabolic pathway that occurs in the absence of insulin. This pathway utilizes an enzyme called aldose reductase which changes glucose into its alcohol form, sorbitol, which accumulates in cells. This compound is very similar to the structure of myoinositol which is necessary for the scavenging of free radicals in cells. Sorbitol inhibits uptake of myoinositol from food due to competitive inhibition and subsequent myoinositol deficiency results in oxidative stress and cellular damage.

Non-enzymatic glycosylation is the third main mechanism of glucose metabolism in an insulin-deficient state and results in an advanced glycosylation end product which cross-links to other proteins and causes stiffening of blood vessels walls. Glycosylation of proteins such as immunoglobulins can inactivate them and affect the body's ability to fight infections.

In addition to microvascular complications of diabetes, macrovascular complications, specifically peripheral artery disease, coronary artery disease, and stroke, also disproportionately affect individuals with diabetes. The theorized mechanism by which patients with diabetes are more greatly affected is that elevated glucose levels affect platelet and fibrin actions which increase thrombosis and delay fibrin removal and subsequently increase risk of coronary thrombosis.

References

1. Giannini C, Caprio SC. Islet function in obese adolescents. Diabetes Obes Metab. 2012;14:40–5.
2. Ziegler AG, Rewers M, Simell O, et al. Seroconversion to multiple islet autoantibodies and risk of progression to diabetes in children. JAMA. 2013;309:2473–9.
3. Coppieters KT, Wiberg A, von Herrath MG. Viral infections and molecular mimicry in type 1 diabetes. APMIS. 2012;120:941–9.
4. Cavallo MG, Fava D, Monetini L, Barone F, Pozzilli P. Cell-mediated immune response to beta casein in recent-onset insulin-dependent diabetes: implications for disease pathogenesis. Lancet. 1996;348:926–8.
5. Norris JM, Barriga K, Klingensmith G, Hoffman M, Eisenbarth GS, Erlich HA, Rewers M. Timing of initial cereal exposure in infancy and risk of islet autoimmunity. JAMA. 2003;290:1713–20.
6. Roche EF, Menon A, Gill D, Hoey H. Clinical presentation of type 1 diabetes. Pediatr Diabetes. 2005;6:75–8.

Diagnosis of Type 1 Diabetes

3

Kelly Joseph, Apoorva Ravindranath Waikar, Stephan Siebel, and Anisha Patel

Type 1 diabetes (T1D) is a chronic condition characterized by absolute insulinopenia secondary to immune-mediated destruction of pancreatic β-cells. T1D has a bimodal age distribution of disease diagnosis. The peaks of onset are in early childhood and adolescence; however, it can manifest itself at any age [1]. Indeed, new-onset T1D is observed throughout adulthood, which is a major reason why the disorder is no longer called juvenile diabetes. Prompt diagnosis and treatment are important to prevent acute and potentially life-threatening complications such as diabetic ketoacidosis (DKA). Unfortunately, DKA remains a very common initial presentation of youth with new-onset T1D.

K. Joseph (✉) · A. R. Waikar · S. Siebel · A. Patel
Yale-New Haven Children's Hospital, Department of Pediatrics, Yale School of Medicine, New Haven, CT, USA
e-mail: kelly.joseph@yale.edu; apoorva.waikar@yale.edu; anisha.patel@yale.edu

W. V. Tamborlane (ed.), *Diabetes in Children and Adolescents*, Contemporary Endocrinology,
https://doi.org/10.1007/978-3-030-64133-7_3

Epidemiology

T1D is one of the most prevalent chronic conditions in childhood, estimated to affect 1 in every 300 children in the United States [2]. Worldwide, 90,000 children are diagnosed with T1D each year, but incidence rates greatly vary by geography. For example, Scandinavian countries, Sardinia, United Kingdom, USA, Canada, and Australia have disproportionately high incidence rates of T1D, whereas, it is relatively rare in Asian countries. Differences in genetic susceptibility and local environmental factors have been proposed as possible explanations for variations in incidence rates. It has also been hypothesized that the peak incidence of T1D during early adolescence is due to increased insulin resistance that is observed during pubertal development in girls and boys with and without diabetes (Fig. 3.1). This would also explain why peak incidence rates during puberty occur earlier in girls than in boys. Thus, the combination of insulin resistance and increasing β-cell dysfunction play key roles in conversion of pre-symptomatic T1D to overt manifestation of T1D symptoms, which can occur over a very short or much longer period of time.

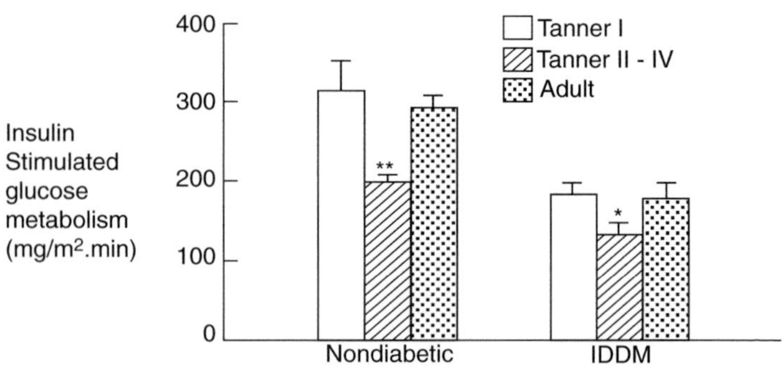

Fig. 3.1 The illustration of insulin resistance of puberty in youth with and without T1D. (From Amiel, et al. NEJM 1986. 315:215–219. Reprinted with permission from the New England Journal of Medicine)

Genetics

As noted in Chap. 2, much work has been done to better understand the genetic background of T1D. A major factor in the pathophysiology of T1D involves autoimmune destruction of β-cells. Two genetic loci have been identified to impart strong genetic susceptibility to developing T1D, that is, major histocompatibility complexes 1 and 2. Both complexes are involved in mediating/regulating immunity and self-recognition. The human MHC is also called the HLA (human leukocyte antigen) complex. HLA class II alleles have been associated with up to 30 to 50% of the overall genetic risk in T1D. The following genetic variants have been found to predispose individuals to an autoimmune reaction against β-cells – HLA DR3/DQ2, HLA-DR4/DQ8, HLA-A*02:01, increased protein tyrosine phosphatase non-receptor type 22 activity, insulin gene polymorphisms, interluekin-2 receptor alpha variants, increased expression of common variant interferon-induced with helicase C domain 1, and mutations on the HLA region of chromosome 6p21. Conversely, genetic variants that are protective against T1D include DRB1*15:01, DQA1*01:02, and DQB1*06:02 [3, 4].

Having a first-degree relative with T1D also is a significant risk factor of developing T1D, as noted in Table 3.1. Within families, inheritance studies have shown an increased risk of T1D in the offspring of fathers with T1D as compared to mothers with T1D [5]. Studies also indicate a higher concordance rate for

Table 3.1 Risk of diabetes in first-degree relatives of individuals with T1D

Group	Childhood annual incidence of T1D
US general population	0.3%
Sibling	3.2%
Mother	2%
Father	4.6%
Both parents	~10%
Dizygotic twin	6%
Monozygotic twin	50%, but incidence varies with age of index twin

monozygotic versus dizygotic twins and an increased sibling risk if one twin is diagnosed at <15 years of age. Further information on the risk of a first-degree relative is provided in the section "Screening for Type 1 Diabetes".

Overall, these gene variants have a low penetrance and are common in Western populations, which may explain why many people do not develop T1D despite having these risk factors. Epigenetic factors, such as DNA methylation and exposure to elevated levels of insulin in utero, are known to influence transcriptional regulation and gene expression, which can account for the variation in concordance rates seen in the siblings. Hence, the development of overt disease is multifactorial and requires both genetic predisposition and environmental triggers.

Diagnosis

The American Diabetes Association classifies diabetes into four categories: (1) T1D – a condition caused by autoimmune destruction of insulin-producing β-cells, (2) type 2 diabetes (T2D) – insulin resistance primarily due to obesity in addition to progressive β-cell dysfunction usually associated with negative autoimmune antibodies, (3) gestational diabetes mellitus – diabetes usually diagnosed in second or third trimester of pregnancy, and (4) other – monogenic types of diabetes, e.g., neonatal diabetes mellitus, maturity-onset diabetes of the young (MODY), disease affecting pancreatic function (e.g., cystic fibrosis–related diabetes, pancreatitis-induced diabetes), and medication-induced diabetes (e.g., glucocorticoids). Nevertheless, this chapter mainly focuses on the diagnosis of T1D, which remains the most common type of diabetes observed in pediatrics.

Typical symptoms which precede the diagnosis of T1D include polyuria, polydipsia, and unintentional weight loss. This can be seen with or without the symptoms of diabetic ketoacidosis including abdominal pain, nausea, vomiting, chest pain, and altered mental status. Most recently, the impact of the COVID-19 virus has been implicated as a potential cause of new onset T1D in pediatrics, but this remains to be determined.

Table 3.2 American Diabetes Association diagnostic criteria for pre-diabetes and diabetes

	Fasting glucose	2-hr glucose during OGTT	HgbA1c	Symptoms
Pre-diabetes	100–125 mg/dL	140–190 mg/dL	5.7–6.4%	Usually asymptomatic
Diabetes	≥126 mg/dL	≥200 mg/dL during OGTT	≥6.5%	Symptoms +random plasma glucose ≥200 mg/dL

Pre-diabetes and T1D can be diagnosed by the specific diagnostic criteria shown in Table 3.2. These criteria include elevated fasting plasma glucose, elevated 2-hour plasma glucose during an oral glucose tolerance test, increased hemoglobin A1c (HbA1c), and/or a random plasma glucose ≥200 mg/dL with or without the symptoms described above. The American Diabetes Association provides guidelines for the diagnosis of diabetes which usually requires at least two of the following: (1) fasting plasma glucose ≥126 mg/dL; (2) two-hour plasma glucose ≥200 mg/dL during oral glucose tolerance test (OGTT); (3) HgbA1c ≥ 6.5%, and 4) random plasma glucose ≥200 mg/dL [6].

Pre-diabetes is a clinical entity in which the glucose levels and HgbA1c are greater than normal but do not meet criteria for diagnosis of diabetes. It is associated with obesity, dyslipidemia, hypertension, and an increased risk for the development of diabetes. Typically, individuals with pre-diabetes progress to T2D; however, it is possible that the labs are reflective of early T1D and they should be repeated based on clinical suspicion and evolution of symptoms.

In the presence of classic signs and symptoms of diabetes, i.e., polyuria, polydipsia, polyphagia, and unintentional weight loss, diabetes can be diagnosed with a single random elevated plasma glucose level ≥200 mg/dL alone. In the absence of unequivocal hyperglycemia, the diagnosis requires two abnormal test results from the same sample or in two separate test samples. If results are equivocal, such as one test meets the diagnostic threshold and the other does not, the positive test should be repeated with a new sample. While c-peptide levels are not included in the diagnostic

Table 3.3 Advantages and disadvantages of various diagnostic testing methods [7]

Testing method	Advantages	Disadvantages
Fasting plasma glucose	Widespread availability, low cost, easy interpretation	Fasting sample required, Reflects glycemia at time of sampling only, influence of acute illness
Oral glucose tolerance test	Most sensitive, earliest marker of glucose dysregulation	Time consuming, fasting required, higher cost, poor reproducibility from day to day
Glycated hemoglobin	Reasonably available across the world with global standardization, marker of long-term glycemia, stable during acute illness, known association of results with complications	Lack of reliability in patients with hemoglobinopathies (e.g., Sickle cell disease and thalassemia), unreliable in anemias with high RBC turnover (e.g., hemolytic anemia) or low RBC turnover (iron deficiency) Lack of reliability after recent transfusion, in advanced renal disease, and between different racial and ethnic populations (higher in African-Americans), higher cost

testing criteria, interpretation of these values can aid in the diagnosis. They can be particularly helpful in distinguishing T1D from T2D where levels would typically be expected to be low and normal to high, respectively.

The advantages and disadvantages of various diagnostic testing methods are shown in Table 3.3 and confounding factors must be considered when interpreting these tests. For example, recent treatment with high-dose glucocorticoids may temporarily increase plasma glucose levels; HbA1c levels may be altered by hemoglobinopathies, anemias, HIV treatment, pregnancy, and race/ethnicity. Disorders associated with increased red blood cell turnover will reflect a lower-than expected HbA1c relative to plasma glucose levels. In these situations, one should consider relying on plasma glucose levels to make the diagnosis. Changes in RBC turnover may adversely affect HbA1c levels in early pregnancy.

T1D can be divided into two categories: immune-mediated and non-autoimmune, idiopathic T1D. The majority of patients fall into the immune-mediated category which is characterized by at least one positive autoantibody out of the four autoantibodies that have been correlated withT1D, and even though not pathogenic, they aid in the diagnosis of T1D. The commonly found autoantibodies target glutamic acid decarboxylase (GAD65), zinc transporter 8 (ZnT8), insulinoma-associated protein type 2 (IA-2), and insulin. Antibodies against GAD65 or insulin are most likely to be the first positive antibodies detected and appear early in life, whereas ZnT8 and IA-2 antibodies are associated with a more rapid progression of symptoms. The presence of more than one autoantibody increases the likelihood of autoimmune T1D. However, a small percentage of the non-diabetic, general population has been found to be positive for one of these autoantibodies, typically GAD65, as well as individuals with T2D.

Some patients will not have detectable antibodies but present with a T1D phenotype. The pathogenesis/etiology of this idiopathic type of diabetes, also referred to as type 1b diabetes, is not fully understood. However, similar to autoimmune-mediated diabetes, T1b leads to absolute insulinopenia. It is distinct from T2D and ketosis-prone (flatbush) diabetes, which is caused by insulin resistance and relative insulinopenia and usually occurs in individuals of African or Asian descent, typically during adulthood. Patients with idiopathic diabetes are prone to ketosis and may have an absolute or intermittent insulin requirement [8, 9]. Table 3.4, adapted from the American Diabetes Association guidelines, outlines a differential diagnosis for classic T1D.

Table 3.4 Differential diagnosis of classic T1D

Type	Anti-islet autoantibodies	Genetics
Classic T1D	Positive >90% of individuals	HLA 30–50% DR3 and DR4 HLA 90% DR3 or DR4 HLA < 3% DQB1*0602
Idiopathic diabetes (T1bD)	Negative	Unknown
T2D	Negative	Unknown
Other	Negative	MODY or other diabetes syndrome

Screening for Type 1 Diabetes

T1DM affects approximately 0.3% of youth <18 years of age in the USA, and the vast majority of patients with T1D do not have a family history of the disease. Results from the TrialNet Study have shed further light on the risk of development of T1D in first-degree relatives. Of the 585 children studied, all of whom are first-degree relatives of individuals with T1DM, 84% of children who were seropositive for two autoantibodies developed T1D compared to 15% of children with single autoantibody positivity and 0.4% in children with no autoantibodies in a 15-year period. There are no currently accepted guidelines regarding screening of relatives of individuals with T1D. Therefore, it is prudent for healthcare providers to be familiar with the symptomology of diabetes and screen for them frequently in patients with first degree relatives with diabetes.

Distinguishing Type 1 from Type 2 Diabetes

Although T1D and T2D have varying pathophysiology, there is a significant clinical overlap which makes the diagnosis at times challenging but essential for determining the right treatment course. The traditional dichotomy of T1DM being a disease of young children and adolescents and T2DM only occurring in the older obese population no longer holds true. Today, we know that both conditions can be diagnosed across all age groups, and due to the current obesity epidemic even patients with T1DM can present with an increased BMI. Furthermore, the presence of DKA at diagnosis, occurring in one-third or more of children with T1D, does not rule out T2DM. DKA is also seen in some individuals with T2D, especially in certain ethnic minorities, such as the Hispanic and Native American populations. Lastly, while T1DM can present at an early age, T2D is rarely seen in children <10 years of age or before onset of puberty. The presence of autoantibodies in conjunction with low C-peptide levels may have diagnostic utility in differentiating patients with T1D from those with T2D.

References

1. Katsarou A, et al. Type 1 diabetes mellitus. Nat Rev Dis Primer. 2017;3:1–19.
2. Hamman RF, et al. The SEARCH for diabetes in youth study: rationale, findings, and future directions. Diabetes Care. 2014;37:3336–44.
3. Eringsmark Regnéll S, Lernmark A. The environment and the origins of islet autoimmunity and type 1 diabetes. Diabet Med. 2013;30:155–60.
4. Pugliese A, et al. HLA-DRB1*15:01-DQA1*01:02-DQB1*06:02 haplotype protects autoantibody-positive relatives. Diabetes. 2016;65:1109–19.
5. Steck AK, Rewers MJ. Genetics of type 1 diabetes. Clin Chem. 2011;57:176–85.
6. American Diabetes Association. Classification and diagnosis of diabetes: standards of medical care in diabetes-2019. Diabetes Care. 2019;42:S13–28.
7. Inzucchi SE. Diagnosis of diabetes. N Engl J Med. 2013;368:192–3.
8. Regnell SE, Lernmark Å. Early prediction of autoimmune (type 1) diabetes. Diabetologia. 2017;60:1370–81.
9. Haaland WC, et al. A-beta-subtype of ketosis-prone diabetes is not predominantly a monogenic diabetic syndrome. Diabetes Care. 2009; 32:873–7.

Initial Management of Youth with Type 1 Diabetes

4

Kerry Stephenson
and William V. Tamborlane

Background

Virtually all of our newly diagnosed patients with type 1 diabetes (T1D) are initially treated with insulin injections. However, the old fashion regimen of pre-breakfast and pre-dinner injections of rapid- and intermediate-acting insulins mixed together in a single syringe has been replaced in most pediatric diabetes treatment centers by multiple daily injection (MDI) regimens that combine long-acting insulin analogs (glargine or detemir) with bolus injections of a rapid-acting insulin analog prior to each meal and large snack. Mixing insulins in a single syringe has also been replaced in many centers by use of insulin pens to administer all insulin injections. Although the first generation of long-acting insulin analogs has been shown to have improved pharmacodynamic profiles for basal insulin replacement compared to prior intermediate acting insulins, they are being replaced by the second generation of ultra-long-acting insulin degludec and U300 glargine. A bio-

K. Stephenson (✉) · W. V. Tamborlane
Yale-New Haven Children's Hospital, Department of Pediatrics,
Yale School of Medicine, New Haven, CT, USA
e-mail: kerry.stephenson@yale.edu; william.tamborlane@yale.edu

W. V. Tamborlane (ed.), *Diabetes in Children and Adolescents*, Contemporary Endocrinology,
https://doi.org/10.1007/978-3-030-64133-7_4

similar U100 glargine, Basaglar, is also available. With basal/bolus MDI regimens, pre-meal bolus doses of first or second generations of rapid-acting insulin analogs are determined by the amount of insulin estimated to be needed to cover the amount of carbohydrate in the meal with corrections for pre-meal blood glucose levels outside the target range, as well as for additional adjustments based on anticipated levels of physical activity following the meal.

While basal/bolus MDI therapy has clear physiologic advantages over traditional NPH-based twice a day (BID) regimens, there are also disadvantages, especially in the treatment of children with new-onset T1D. The flat time-action profiles of long-acting insulins put a premium on compliance with taking bolus doses of rapid-acting insulins with every meal and substantial snack. The number of daily injections is increased further because labeled instructions and recent pharmacodynamic studies indicate that long-acting insulins should be given as separate injections and not mixed with rapid-acting analogs [1]. In addition, calculation of pre-meal bolus doses of rapid-acting insulins requires a degree of experience and expertise that is difficult to teach at the onset of T1D in children and their parents who are overwhelmed by the trauma of learning that diabetes is now part of their daily lives. Moreover, the common occurrence of the partial remission phase of T1D within the first few weeks of initiating insulin therapy makes it possible to achieve target glucose and A1c levels during the early stages of T1D with simplified insulin regimens.

Over the past few years, our Pediatric Type 1 Diabetes Treatment Team has utilized a modified twice-daily insulin regimen of NPH and rapid-acting insulin analog in the morning and rapid-acting insulin analog and insulin detemir at dinner for patients with new-onset T1D. The rationale for this approach was that the relatively flat and consistent insulin profile of the pre-dinner detemir would lower the risk of nocturnal hypoglycemia compared to pre-dinner NPH or even pre-dinner or bedtime glargine. Moreover, the pre-breakfast injection of NPH insulin (in combination with the patient's residual endogenous insulin secretion) obviates the need for extra insulin to cover lunch and afternoon snacks. Since the pre-dinner dose of detemir may not last the full 24 hours, the morning dose of NPH insulin can also cover the waning effects of detemir before dinner. Consequently, most of our patients can achieve and maintain good glycemic control for the initial 3 to 6 months of "old fashion" treatment (Fig. 4.1). It is also why we have called this period "The Bridge to Insulin Pump Treatment." Indeed, once patients/parents have obtained experience with management of diabetes at home and glycemic control becomes more difficult due to the progressive loss of residual endogenous insulin secretion after 6 months, patients are switched to a basal/bolus regimen, which in our practice almost always involves continuous subcutaneous insulin infusion (CSII) pump therapy (Fig. 4.1).

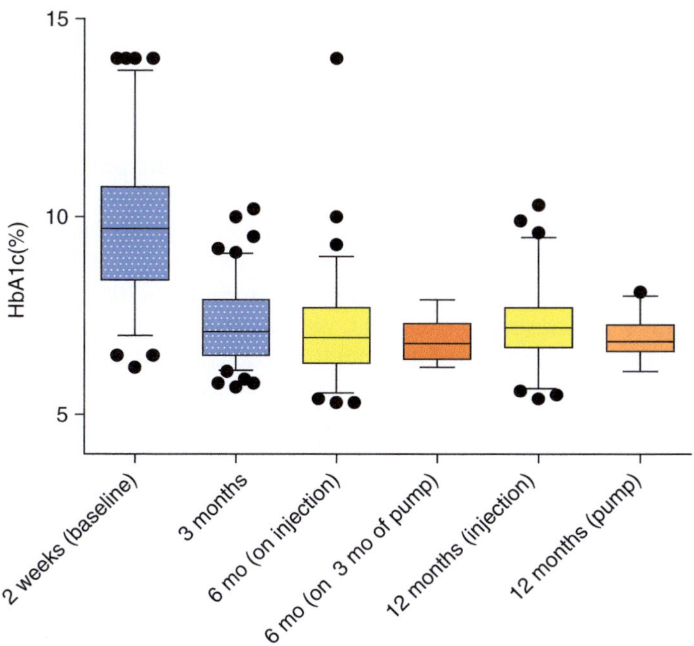

Fig. 4.1 HbA1c% levels expressed as median (25%, 75%) at 3, 6, and 12 months for children with T1D within the first year of diagnosis grouped by the type of insulin treatment. (Reprinted from Endocrine Practice (Ref. [2] below) with permission)

Initial Treatment Regimen

Almost all of our patients with newly diagnosed T1D are admitted to the Yale-New Haven Children's Hospital for initiation of insulin treatment and diabetes education. While there have been several studies that support initial outpatient treatment of youth with new-onset T1D, our experience suggests that an initial hospital admission even for only 1–3 days allows parents to adjust to the diagnosis of T1D in their child in an environment that they perceive as safe. It was noteworthy that more of our patients have received initial outpatient treatment during the Covid-19 pandemic, due in part to the perception that the hospital was no longer a safe environment. The support that our Children's Hospital provides for a "Diabetes Specialist" who is responsible for initial diabetes education has also been very well received by our families in both the inpatient and the outpatient settings.

Twice-daily insulin injections are started either on admission to the hospital or following correction of DKA, usually with a total daily dose (TDD) of insulin of 0.5–1.0 units per kg body weight. The starting insulin doses are divided as follows: separate pen injections of NPH (40% of TDD) and rapid-acting insulin analog (~20% of TDD) at breakfast and separate injections of rapid analog (~20% of TDD) and detemir insulin (~20% TDD) at dinner. At the start of treatment, patients and parents learn basic diabetes management skills with a special emphasis on learning how to count the carbohydrate content of meals. During the initial 2–3 weeks of treatment, insulin doses are titrated toward target pre-meal glucose values of 80–130 mg/dl during daily telephone contacts with the Diabetes Specialist. During the early insulin dose titration period, parents and patients are encouraged to maintain a relatively fixed carbohydrate intake with each meal. During follow-up clinic visits (approximately 2, 6, 13, 26, 39, and 52 weeks following diagnosis), glycemic control is assessed by review of self-monitoring of blood glucose (SMBG) records and by point-of-service A1c measurements; episodes of severe hypoglycemia, re-admissions for DKA, and changes in insulin regimens are also recorded. It is also noteworthy that an increasing proportion of our patients have been starting to use current generations of continuous glucose monitors (CGM) to replace blood glucose meter monitoring very early in the course of their diabetes. Indeed, CGM is typically ordered at the initial follow-up office visit, 1 to 2 weeks after discharge from the hospital. The concepts of correction doses and insulin to carbohydrate ratios that enable more flexible carbohydrate intake are introduced during the second or third follow-up clinic visits.

Families are also encouraged to switch to continuous subcutaneous insulin infusion (CSII) insulin pump therapy as soon as they are ready, especially in very young patients who often require small total daily doses of insulin, as well as very small correction doses. Educational materials regarding pump therapy are provided during initial diabetes education, and approximately 30% or more of families in our practice switch to pump therapy after less than 3 months of injection therapy. In other patients, the decision to switch to CSII occurs later, commonly due to increasing difficulties in maintaining adequate glycemic control during the second half of the first year of treatment of T1D. It is often challenging to receive insurance coverage for insulin pump therapy in patients whose diabetes is <6 months duration. A negative aspect of initial treatment with twice-daily insulin injections is that some families are very reluctant to switch to full basal/bolus treatment given by either an insulin pump or multiple daily injections.

Clinical Outcomes During the First Year of Treatment

As we reported more than 10 years ago, approximately half of our patients were using basal/bolus treatment for their diabetes by the end of the first year of treatment [2]. In those patients, the median total daily insulin doses at 3, 6, and 12 months were 0.6, 0.7 and 0.8 u/kg/day, respectively, and nadir A1c levels were observed at 6 months (i.e., 6.8 to 6.9%). By 12 months, patients who had switched to pump therapy had a median A1c of 6.9% compared to 7.2% in injection patients. There were severe hypoglycemic events in only 5% of patients during the first year of treatment; all occurred with injection therapy during daytime, and all but one of the patients was younger than 7 years of age. None of the patients had an episode of DKA during the first year of treatment.

Conclusions

Very effective glycemic control can be achieved in youth with new-onset T1D during the first 3 to 6 months of treatment using a modified BID regimen that employs a long-acting insulin analog rather than NPH insulin for overnight basal insulin replacement. This simplified regimen provides time for families to acquire experience in basic management skills, as well as to learn advanced management concepts, including insulin to carbohydrate ratios and correction doses. Consequently, patients and parents are well prepared to switch to CSII by 3 months if this approach to insulin replacement is preferred by the families. It is also noteworthy that a clinical advantage of the modified BID regimen is the low frequency of clinical and biochemical hypoglycemia, especially low glucose levels during the night. Indeed, the rationale for choosing detemir in this regimen is based on studies in adults and children with T1D that indicate greater within-subject consistency in pharmacodynamic responses of detemir versus glargine [3, 4].

It is important to emphasize that we are not suggesting that the injection regimen that we have employed as initial therapy is superior to initial basal/bolus therapy given as either CSII or MDI in youth at onset of T1D. Rather, a BID regimen that employs morning NPH insulin and a night time long-acting insulin analog combined with a morning and dinner rapid-acting insulin analog remains an effective option for initial treatment that can yield best clinical outcomes that have been reported to date with basal/bolus therapy. Nevertheless, an increasing percentage of families are choosing initial basal/bolus therapy using multiple daily injections, since adding a third dose of rapid-acting insulin at lunchtime allows for greater variability in carbohydrate intake with this meal.

As noted previously, it is now common for families to use current generations of CGM devices within weeks of diagnosis of diabetes as a replacement for blood glucose meter monitoring and as a method for remote monitoring of sensor glucose levels. New and improved integrated CGM/insulin pump closed-loop systems have already been approved for use in the treatment of T1D. Best of all, the new integrated CGM and pump systems promise improved clinical outcomes with a reduced burden of treatment in parents and their children with T1D. It should also be noted that aggressive MDI treatment with insulin injections and/or insulin pumps can provide persistent reductions in HbA1c levels that are similar to that which can be currently achieved with recent advances in diabetes technology (Fig. 4.2).

We have also included a copy of the treatment manual that we are using for initial education of families with a child with new-onset T1D in the Appendix of this book.

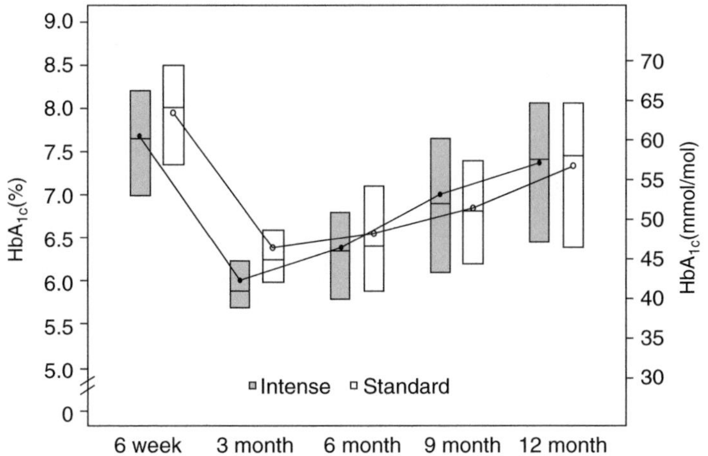

Fig. 4.2 No differences in A1c in the Intensive and Standard treatment groups during first 12 months of treatment. (Re-printed with permission from Diabetes Care (Ref. [5] below))

References

1. Cengiz E, Tamborlane WV, Martin-Fredericksen M, Dziura J, Weinzimer SA. Early pharmacokinetic and pharmacodynamic effects of mixing lispro with glargine insulin: results of glucose clamp studies in youth with type 1 diabetes. Diabetes Care. 2010;33:1009–12.
2. Cengiz E, Sherr JL, Sikes K, Urban A, Weinzimer SA. Tamborlane WV for the Yale Pediatric Type 1 Diabetes Treatment Team. A bridge to insulin pump therapy: BID regimen with NPH and detemir insulin during initial treatment of youth with type 1 diabetes. Endocr Pract. 2011;6:1–17.
3. Heise T, Nosek L, Ronn BB, et al. Lower within-subject variability of insulin detemir in comparison to NPH insulin and insulin glargine in people with type 1 diabetes. Diabetes. 2004;53:1614–20.
4. Danne T, Lupke K, Walte K, Von Schuetz W, Gall MA. Insulin detemir is characterized by a consistent pharmacokinetic profile across age-groups in children, adolescents, and adults with type 1 diabetes. Diabetes Care. 2003;26:3087–92.
5. Diabetes Research in Children Network (DirecNet) and Type 1 Diabetes TrialNet Study Groups. Effectiveness of early intensive therapy on Beta cell preservation in type 1 diabetes. Diabetes care. Diabetes Care. 2013;36:4030–5.

5 Insulin Treatment of Type 1 Diabetes

Eda Cengiz, Michelle Van Name,
and William V. Tamborlane

Background

The discovery of insulin in 1921 transformed type 1 diabetes (T1D) from a death sentence to a chronic disease with a demanding treatment regimen. Prior to the advent of insulin, the life expectancy of children with T1D was approximately 1 year from diagnosis. Leonard Thompson, a teenager with T1DM, has been reported to be the first patient treated with insulin by Banting, Best, Collip, and Macleod in 1922 [1]. Since then, insulin has become one of the best-characterized hormones, with a wealth of data on its crystalline structure and mechanism of action at the molecular, cellular, and organ levels. Its chemical structure was determined in 1951 which paved the way for insulin's chemical

E. Cengiz (✉) · M. Van Name · W. V. Tamborlane
Yale-New Haven Children's Hospital, Department of Pediatrics,
Yale School of Medicine, New Haven, CT, USA
e-mail: eda.cengiz@yale.edu; michelle.vanname@yale.edu

W. V. Tamborlane (ed.), *Diabetes in Children and Adolescents*, Contemporary Endocrinology,
https://doi.org/10.1007/978-3-030-64133-7_5

synthesis in 1960. The three-dimensional structure was determined by Dorothy Hodgkin in 1969, the insulin gene was cloned in 1980, and recombinant human insulin has been available commercially since that time. Most recently, insulin therapy has been transformed by the introduction of amino acid substitutions in the human insulin molecule that have produced more rapid- and long-acting insulin analogs compared to human insulin formulations.

Insulin Action and Secretion

Insulin plays a central role in the regulation of carbohydrate, lipid, and protein metabolism in humans, as well as other vertebrate species. In healthy, non-diabetic individuals, low basal insulin levels regulate hepatic glycogenolysis resulting in fasting glucose production rates of ~2 mg/kg/minute in adults and between 5 and 7 mg/kg/minute in young children. As soon as insulin levels rise after meals, hepatic glucose production is suppressed and glycogenesis and fatty acid synthesis are enhanced. In muscle, insulin's main function is to facilitate glucose entry into the cell by binding to the insulin receptor, which then upregulates GLUT4. Once inside muscle, glucose is used for immediate energy expenditure, as well as for building glycogen stores. Hence, the concept of carbohydrate loading prior to track meets and other physical activities by elite athletes.

Insulin also promotes positive nitrogen balance by enhancing amino acid uptake, inhibiting protein breakdown, and promoting protein synthesis. Insulin secretion after carbohydrate intake is a highly dynamic process regulated by various factors, although glucose is the main stimulator of insulin release from the β-cell. Insulin release occurs in a characteristic biphasic pattern – an acute "first phase" that lasts only a few minutes, followed by a sustained "second phase" of insulin secretion; half-maximal stimulation of insulin occurs at about 144 mg/dL. Insulin is secreted directly into the portal vein and is immediately degraded by liver insulinases to approximately half of its original concentration. In serum, insulin levels rise to maximum levels 30 to 45 minutes after food ingestion and decline to basal levels by 2 to 3 hours after meals. Although glucose is the strongest stimulator of insulin secretion, other sugars (e.g., mannose), certain amino acids (e.g., arginine and leucine), GLP1, other hormones and neurotransmitters, and vagal nerve stimulation also modulate insulin secretion, keeping glucose concentrations in a narrow range.

Insulin Treatment of Type 1 Diabetes

Although near normoglycemia has been a goal of treatment of T1D since the successful completion of the Diabetes Control and Complications Trial, clinical use of insulin is remarkably complex and optimal metabolic control is very difficult to achieve and maintain. With so many nutritional, hormonal, and lifestyle variables affecting glucose homeostasis, there is rarely a predictable treatment regimen that applies to all patients at all times, especially in children and adolescents with T1D. Indeed, in youth with T1D, treatment regimens remain under constant scrutiny warranting regular reassessments and fine-tuning. The inconvenient truth is that no insulin treatment regimen will ever be perfect until there is feedback control of insulin delivery based on real-time measurements of sensor glucose levels. Fortunately, new, semi-automatic hybrid closed-loop insulin delivery systems are beginning to meet that need.

Animal and Human Insulin Preparations

Shortly after the discovery of insulin, pork and beef insulin products became the treatment of choice for many decades. In early commercial production, trace quantities of zinc were added to produce "regular" insulin, a more stable (crystalline zinc) insulin preparation [2]. The duration of regular insulin was on average 5 to 8 hours, often too short for overnight glucose control and too long acting when injected in large doses before meals. In fact, it was subsequently shown that large doses of regular insulin injected before dinner contributed to episodes of nocturnal hypoglycemia many hours later. In 1946, Dr. Hans Christian Hagedorn's laboratory produced a protamine zinc insulin, which became known as NPH (neutral protamine Hagedorn) insulin. Another method to prolongate insulin action was the creation of a zinc–insulin complex in the presence of an acetate buffer. This insulin could be produced in a completely crystalline form (ultralente) or as an amorphous precipitate (semilente). The combination of these two zinc-acetate insulins (70% ultralente and 30% semilente) created lente insulin, with a similar duration of action as NPH insulin. One of the major limitations of these animal insulins was their immunogenic potential, due to impurities in pancreatic extracts.

Current Basal/Bolus Regimens Using Insulin Analogs

The first synthesis of human insulin by recombinant DNA (rDNA) technology in 1978 represents a seminal milestone in the history of insulin, since it enabled the production of virtually unlimited quantities of human insulin. Even more important, rDNA technology paved the way for the production of insulin analogs with rapid-acting and long-acting pharmacokinetics (PK) and pharmacodynamics (PD).

Rapid-Acting Insulin Analogs Rapid-acting insulin analogs (RAIs) were the first modified human insulin preparations. In these analogs, human insulin was modified by changing the amino acid sequence that increases the rate of absorption from the subcutaneous tissue. Changes in amino acid sequences, e.g., replacement of proline by lysine at B28 and lysine by proline at B29, led to the development of *insulin lispro* [3]. The second rapid-acting insulin analog, *insulin aspart*, was produced by replacing proline by aspartic acid at B28. The PK/PD time-action curves of both of these insulin analogs are very similar. The third rapid-acting insulin analog, *insulin glulisine*, was developed by replacing asparagine with lysine at B3 and replacing lysine with glutamic acid at B29. These changes in the ß-chain of human insulin impaired the tendency of insulin molecules to form tightly aggregated insulin hexamers, resulting in faster dissociation in the subcutaneous space after injection.

These new rapid insulin analogs (RIAs) reduced postprandial glucose excursions as compared to regular insulin due to their more rapid time-action profiles. These RIAs permitted insulin injections closer to meal onset, allowing greater flexibility in daily life. Moreover, the risk of late post-meal hypoglycemia was also reduced. Insulin lispro and aspart are also the insulins of choice for use in continuous subcutaneous insulin infusion pumps, where algorithms for bolus calculation and basal rate adaptations rely on the more rapid onset of action of these insulins. Faster onset of action, earlier peak activity, and higher peak concentrations of RIAs have been particularly beneficial in overcoming problems associated with insulin resistance of puberty.

Insulin lispro was the first rapid-acting insulin analog approved by the FDA for clinical use. Studies comparing regular insulin and insulin lispro demonstrated no difference in affinity to the insulin receptor. Clinical trials have demonstrated that insulin lispro acts within 15 minutes, peaks at approximately 1 hour, and lasts 3 to 5 hours after subcutaneous injection.

Insulin aspart was approved for clinical use in the United States in June 2000. Preclinical studies have shown that the insulin aspart has the same insulin receptor and IGF-1 receptor interaction kinetics as human insulin, diminishing concerns about its mitogenic potential [4, 5]. Similar to insulin lispro, insulin aspart was conceptualized as a meal-time insulin. It is absorbed more rapidly than human regular insulin, reaches higher maximal concentrations sooner, and has a shorter duration of action. In a multicenter study, the risk of postprandial hypoglycemia requiring third-party intervention was reduced significantly without leading to deterioration of late postprandial blood glucose levels when insulin aspart was compared to regular insulin.

Insulin glulisine has a similar pharmacokinetic, pharmacodynamic, and safety profile as compared to other rapid-acting insulin analogs and is formulated without the addition of zinc. It does not appear to accumulate in patients with renal impairment. Insulin glulisine is comparable to other rapid-acting analogs with respect to glycemic control, and its somewhat faster absorption rate has questionable clinical significance.

In most diabetes centers, insulin lispro, aspart, and glulisine are used interchangeably when it comes to selecting a rapid-acting insulin for either Continuus Subcutaneous Insulin Infusion (CSII) or as part of multiple-daily injection regimens. However, glulisine insulin has been shown to increase the frequency of catheter occlusions when used in insulin pumps. Conversely, we have shown that there is earlier peak and shorter duration of action with increasing duration of infusion site use with both insulin lispro and insulin aspart [6] (Fig. 5.1). Moreover, randomized, multicenter studies in pregnant women with T1D found insulin lispro and insulin aspart to be safe for mother and offspring. Congenital abnormalities do not appear to be more frequent with either lispro or aspart use during pregnancy. As noted above, in a comparison clamp study of insulin lispro and insulin aspart, we were unable to detect any PK or PD differences with these two rapid-acting insulin analogs [6].

Ultra-Rapid-Acting Insulin Analogs While near-normal post-meal glycemic control can be achieved by RIAs, the limitations of these early, rapid-acting insulin analogs have become more apparent as tight glycemic control has been accepted as standard of care diabetes. Even faster onset and offset of insulin action, replicating physiologic insulin action, is needed to provide better glycemic control, minimize hypoglycemic episodes, and reduce weight gain. A number of new insulin analogs have already been approved that aim to achieve faster insulin action.

- *Ultra-rapid-acting insulin aspart* (Fiasp; Novo Nordisk) is insulin aspart with new excipients (nicotinamide and L-asparaginase) that result in faster initial absorption after SC injection. Compared with insulin aspart, Fiasp is associated with a faster onset of action and increased early exposure that, in turn, leads to a significantly greater early glucose-lowering effect. Furthermore, increased early exposure with faster-acting insulin aspart led to improved glycemic control following a post-meal challenge without an increase in hypoglycemia.

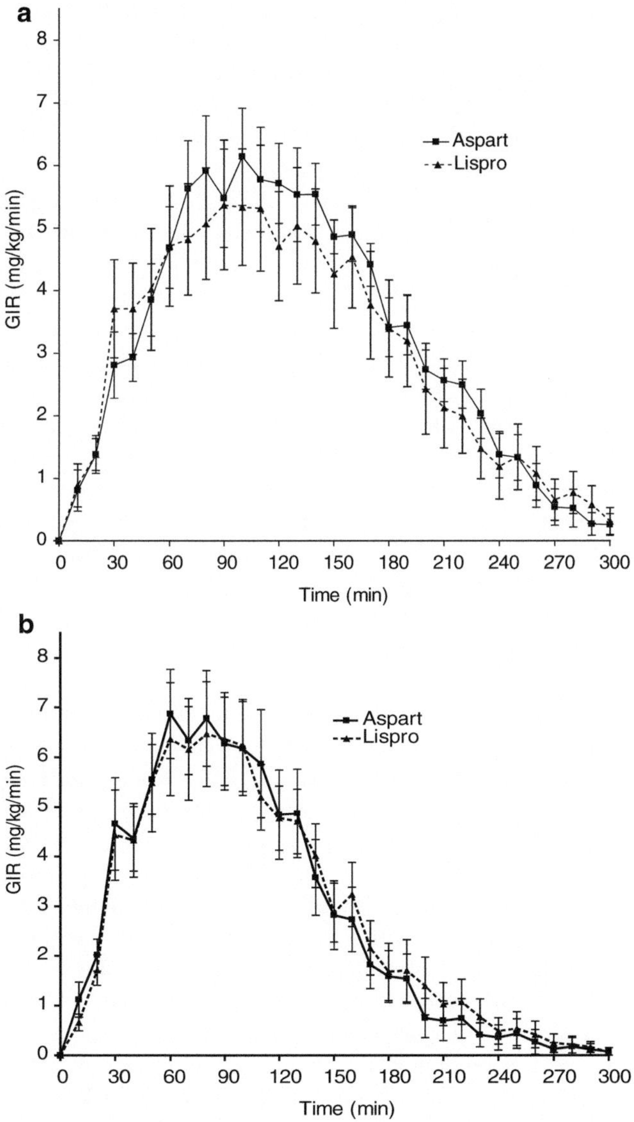

Fig. 5.1 Pharmacodynamic profiles. Insulin action, expressed as GIR required to maintain euglycemia after standard bolus of 0.2 unit/kg insulin aspart or lispro. Data presented as mean ± SEM. (**a**) Day 1 of catheter site insertion. (**b**) Day 4 of catheter site insertion. (From Swan, et al. (Ref. [6]) with permission)

- *Ultra-rapid-acting lispro* was developed by adding excipients (citrate and treprostinil) to the original insulin lispro formulation. With this agent, insulin absorption from the subcutaneous tissue is more rapid due to by citrate's effect on increasing vascular permeability and treprostinil's effect on enhancing local vasodilatation at the injection site.
- *Afrezza, inhaled insulin,* may be the fastest acting exogenous insulin, since its insulin is absorbed quickly by inhalation, eliminating the delays after subcutaneous injection. Afrezza insulin is delivered by a thumb-sized inhaler specifically designed for its delivery to the large surface area of the lungs. Once inhaled, Afrezza dissolves rapidly in the alveolar fluid of the lungs and is rapidly absorbed into systemic circulation. Afrezza insulin was approved for treating adult patients with T1DM and T2DM by the FDA in 2014, and clinical studies are underway for use in pediatric diabetes. Afrezza is contraindicated in patients with asthma or chronic obstructive pulmonary disease, and it is not recommended for patients who smoke. Basic spirometry testing should be done to assess FEV1 at baseline, after 6 months of therapy and annually, thereafter, even in the absence of pulmonary symptoms.

Long-Acting Insulin Analogs At the other end of the pharmacodynamic spectrum, the first long-acting basal insulin analog, *insulin glargine*, was developed to create prolonged and peakless PK/PD profile by precipitation of soluble glargine at the site of injection and slow release of insulin into the circulation. This analog resulted from the elongation of the β-chain at position 30 by two arginine residues as well as by substitution of asparagine at the 21 position of the α-chain with glycine to maintain chemical stability. Consequently, insulin glargine is soluble in solution in the weakly acid pH of its excipients and precipitates in neutral pH. When insulin glargine is injected into the subcutaneous tissue (neutral pH), it precipitates, slowing and stabilizing the absorption of this peakless insulin. Insulin glargine was initially reported to have a flat profile; however, more recent studies demonstrate a gentle rise in effect with a modest peak at 6 hours and a duration of action of ~24 hours. A major clinical benefit of this peakless basal insulin, especially for pediatric use, is the potential reduction of nocturnal hypoglycemia.

Insulin detemir was created by attaching a myristic acid to B-29 and removing threonine from B-30 of human insulin molecule to slow adsorption and facilitate extended plasma circulation through non-covalent albumin binding. These molecular changes enhance albumin binding once detemir insulin is injected subcutaneously leading to a slow absorption from the site and prolongation of insulin action in the circulation. Its biological duration of action is dose dependent lasting between 12 and 24 hours. It has less intrasubject insulin variability of absorption and better reproducibility than glargine insulin [7]. Insulin detemir acts in the brain as well as in the peripheral tissue, which might lead to appetite suppression that can explain some of the reduced weight gain observed during treatment with detemir. However, twice a day injections of insulin detemir seem to be more common when used in children and adolescents with T1D.

In order to reduce the number of daily injections for children and adolescents with T1D, many pediatric endocrinologists mixed rapid-acting and long-acting insulins in a single syringe. However, we have shown that such mixing is not recommended since it markedly delays the absorption of the rapid-acting component of that mixture (Fig. 5.2) [8].

Ultra-Long-Acting Insulin Analogs Ultra-long-acting insulins are defined as insulins with a glucose lowering effect beyond 24 hours after subcutaneous injection. Ultra-long-acting insulins have been developed to mitigate the injection burden and to improve treatment compliance. Ultra-long-acting profiles coupled with lower day-to-day within-subject variability and peakless insulin action have been key targets for ultra-long-acting insulin formulations.

- *Insulin glargine U300* is an ultra-long-acting insulin that has been approved for use in T1D and T2D. It delivers the same dose of glargine in one-third of the volume with a more prolonged pharmacokinetic and pharmacodynamic profile than

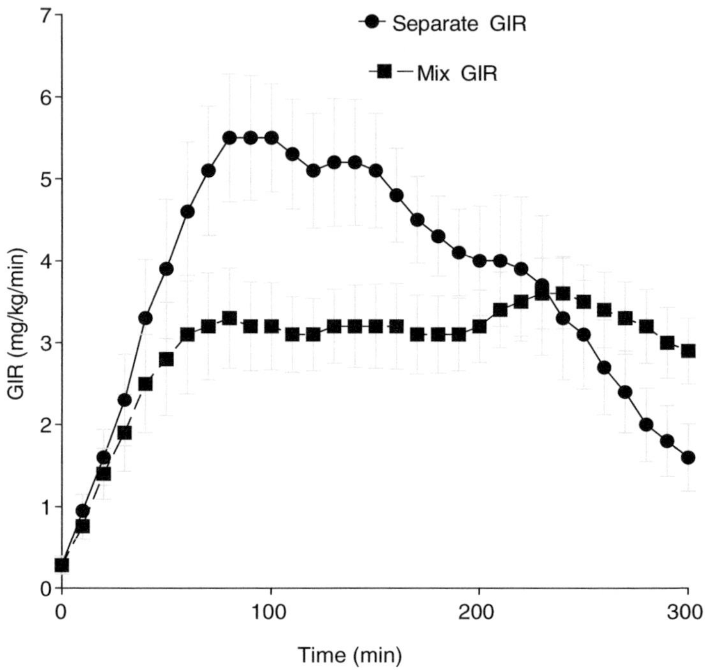

Fig. 5.2 Pharmacodynamics of insulin aspart and insulin detemir given as separated injection compared to a single mixed injection. (From Cengiz et al. [8], with permission)

glargine U100. Glargine U300 is released more gradually from the subcutaneous tissue, giving it a more constant pharmacokinetic profile with a less pronounced peak of action and low within-day and low between-day variability.

- *Insulin degludec* is an ultra-long-acting basal insulin with a modified structure that leads to the formation of multihexamers upon subcutaneous injection, resulting in a depot from which IDeg is released very slowly and continuously into the circulation [7]. It reversibly binds to serum protein albumin, resulting in a relatively high concentration of insulin degludec in the bloodstream that contributes to its prolonged kinetics. The daily injected dose reaches steady state after 2–3 days of once-daily administration [9]. Insulin degludec has a 42-hour duration of action with an even distribution of glucose-lowering activity and a terminal half-life of 25–26 hours once steady state is achieved. It has been shown to have a lower day-to-day within-subject variability and similar effect on HbA1c and weight reduction compared with glargine 100. Our clinical experience indicates that switching from glargine or detemir to degludec lowered A1C levels in youngsters with T2D but not T1D [10].

References

1. Bliss M. Banting's, Best's, and Collip's accounts of the discovery of insulin. Bull Hist Med. 1982;56:554–68.
2. Scott DA. Crystalline insulin. Biochem J. 1934;1592-1602(1591):28.
3. Howey DC, Bowsher RR, Brunelle RL, Woodworth JR. [Lys(B28), Pro(B29)]-human insulin. A rapidly absorbed analogue of human insulin. Diabetes. 1994;43:396–402.
4. Lindholm A, McEwen J, Riis AP. Improved postprandial glycemic control with insulin aspart. A randomized double-blind cross-over trial in type 1 diabetes. Diabetes Care. 1999;22:801–5.
5. Mudaliar SR, Lindberg FA, Joyce M, et al. Insulin aspart (B28 asp-insulin): a fast-acting analog of human insulin: absorption kinetics and action profile compared with regular human insulin in healthy nondiabetic subjects. Diabetes Care. 1999;22:1501–6.
6. Swan KL, Dziura JD, Steil GM, Voskanyan GR, Sikes KA, Steffen AT, Martin ML, Tamborlane WV, Weinzimer SA. Effect of age of infusion site and type of rapid-acting insulin analog on the pharmacodynamic and pharmacokinetic parameters in youth with T1DM on insulin pump therapy. Diabetes Care. 2009;32:240–4.
7. Heinemann L, Sinha K, Weyer C, Loftager M, Hirschberger S, Heise T. Time-action profile of the soluble, fatty acid acylated, long-acting insulin analogue NN304. Diabet Med. 1999;16:332–8.
8. Cengiz E, Swan KL, Tamborlane WV, Sherr JL, Fredericksen-Martin M, Weinzimer SA. The alteration of Aspart insulin pharmacodynamics (PD) when mixed with Detemir insulin. Diabetes Care. 2012;35:690–2.
9. Heise T, Korsatko S, Nosek L, et al. Steady state is reached within 2-3 days of once-daily administration of degludec, a basal insulin with an ultralong duration of action. J Diabetes. 2016;8:132–8.
10. Elahi S, Patel A, Guandalini C, Steffen A, Sherr J, Tamborlane WV, Van Name M. Impact of switching youth with diabetes to insulin degludec in clinical practice. Endocr Pract. 2019;25:226–9.

Insulin Pump Therapy

6

Elizabeth A. Doyle, Eda Cengiz,
and William V. Tamborlane

Background

Continuous subcutaneous insulin infusion (CSII), commonly referred as insulin pump treatment, was introduced more than 40 years ago [1]. At the dawn of the era of intensive treatment of T1D, we reasoned that use of a pump device that was able to deliver regular insulin as a continuous basal infusion combined with the ability to deliver larger boluses of insulin before mealtime could simulate the physiologic fluctuations in plasma insulin seen in children without diabetes. While the delayed peak and longer duration of action of the pre-meal bolus of regular insulin made it impossible to fully normalize meal-related patterns of insulin secretion, the ability to give separate bolus doses tailored to the carbohydrate content of each meal would allow much better control of post-meal hyperglycemia. Moreover, we theorized that

E. A. Doyle (✉)
Yale School of Nursing, Primary Care Division, Orange, CT, USA
e-mail: elizabeth.doyle@yale.edu

E. Cengiz · W. V. Tamborlane
Yale-New Haven Children's Hospital, Department of Pediatrics,
Yale School of Medicine, New Haven, CT, USA
e-mail: Eda.Cengiz@yale.edu

W. V. Tamborlane (ed.), *Diabetes in Children and Adolescents*, Contemporary Endocrinology,
https://doi.org/10.1007/978-3-030-64133-7_6

the delayed fall in plasma glucose several hours after the meal would be minimized by endogenous counter-regulatory hormone defense mechanisms. A single basal infusion rate was perceived to be sufficient and that stable plasma insulin levels during the overnight period would be relatively easy to accomplish with the continuous subcutaneous insulin infusion. In comparison to what was then being achieved with conventional injections of insulin, improvements in glycemic control in the initial inpatient and outpatient insulin pump studies were spectacular (Fig. 6.1) [2, 3]. Moreover, the demonstration that the subcutaneous route of insulin administration was not as great a barrier to effective treatment as had been previously perceived, paved the way for the develop-

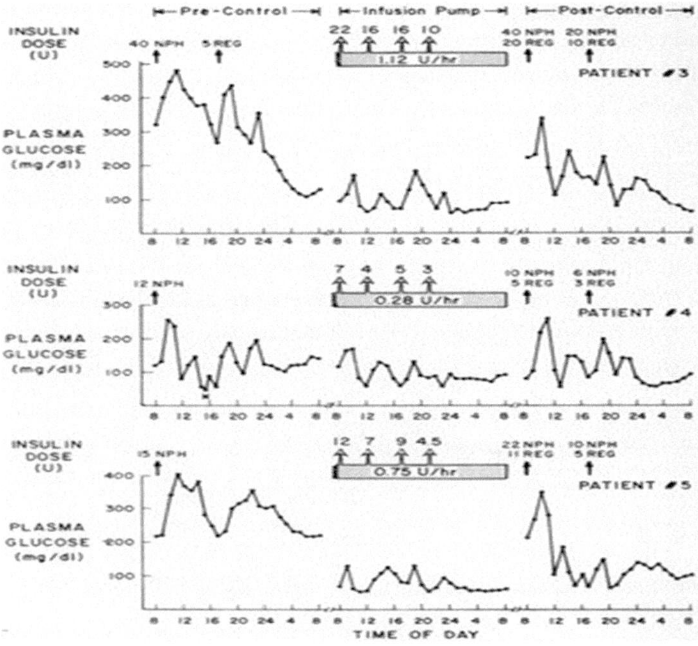

Fig. 6.1 Blood glucose profiles in three patients in the first successful insulin pump study (versus pre- and post-control). (From: Tamborlane et al. NEJM 1979; 300:573–578)

ment of similar basal/bolus approaches using multiple daily injections of insulin (MDI).

Today's Insulin Pumps

Most of today's insulin pumps are composed of an insulin reservoir that is incorporated into a programmable insulin delivery device. In most traditional pumps, plastic tubing connects the insulin reservoir to a catheter that is inserted subcutaneously into either the abdomen or hip. Tubeless insulin pumps (AKA patch pumps) have slightly different structures that are directly connected to the subcutaneous tissue through a catheter without any tubing. Typically, patch pumps require that signals from a hand-handheld device be communicated to the pump via a wireless link to enable adjustments in insulin dose settings.

The pump is programmed to deliver "basal rates" of rapid-acting insulin throughout the day; rates that can be programmed to change up to 48 times during a 24-hour period. Variations in basal rate can be particularly beneficial overnight, since basal rates can be programmed to decrease in the early part of the night to prevent hypoglycemia and increased in the hours before dawn to keep glucose from rising. Nevertheless, prior to the introduction of continuous glucose monitoring, few families checked nocturnal glucose levels very often. Basal rates also eliminate the need for the use of intermediate or long-acting insulins, and meal planning does not have to center around peaking insulin action, as recommended with multiple daily injection therapy.

During the day, the patient "dials up" a bolus of rapid-acting insulin in accordance with the carbohydrate content of the meal. This allows more flexibility in the quantity and content of food intake. Unfortunately, many patients and parents are not particularly skilled in calculating the carbohydrate content of meals. This observation points to the importance of continued education from both the registered dietitian and the diabetes provider.

Some of the limitations of insulin pumps are possible encumbrance during exercise or contact sports. While the pumps with tubing can be removed for a short period of time during such sports, it takes careful planning and close monitoring before, during, and after the exercise period. Additionally, because only rapid-acting insulin is used, any interruption in flow (catheter occlusion or disconnection) can lead to relatively rapid deterioration of metabolic control, especially during sleeping hours. Although uncommon, local infections at the site of catheter insertion can occur, especially if improper hygienic technique is employed or site changes are delayed.

It also is important for families to understand that insulin pump therapy is costly. A recent Swedish study demonstrated that mean annual costs were higher for adults with T1D (in Sweden) who used insulin pumps versus those who used multiple daily injection therapy ($12,928 vs. $9005, respectively) [4]. Thus, it is essential that families investigate their health care insurance coverage and out-of-pocket costs to ensure that they have the financial means for this treatment choice.

Insulin pumps emerged as an ideal tool to intensify insulin treatment while minimizing hypoglycemia in the 1980s. However, very few pediatric patients initially used these devices because they were cumbersome to use, few pediatric providers had experience in the use of pumps and there was uncertainty about the long-term benefits of intensive treatment. The results of the Diabetes Control and Complications Trial (DCCT) indicating that the long-term benefits of strict diabetes control outweigh the risks of severe hypoglycemia resulted in a major paradigm shift in diabetes treatment [5]. As a result, intensive diabetes management rapidly became the gold standard, and insulin pump therapy was promoted by expert diabetes care providers as an effective means of achieving strict metabolic control of T1D. For example, very few patients used insulin pumps during the early days of the DCCT study, but this increased to >40% of intensively treated patients by the end of the study. Moreover, many improvements in pump therapy have led to advanced pump features including multiple programmable basal/bolus rates and correction factors (AKA the sensitivity factor), ability to adjust basal and bolus doses in small increments, bolus history functions to assess missing bolus doses of insulin, and the incorporation of mini-computers to calculate mealtime and correction doses of insulin. As a result, the

T1D Exchange Registry of patients in the United States has recently reported that HbA1c levels are consistently lower in patients using insulin pump therapy than in patients on multiple daily injection regimens [6].

Identifying Pediatric Pump Candidates

While insulin pump therapy has been demonstrated to be effective in the management of T1D, not all pediatric patients make good pump candidates. When considering whether or not to initiate insulin pump therapy, it is essential that care providers select candidates and families in whom pump therapy would be both safe and effective. Indications for pump therapy in pediatrics include persistently elevated A1c levels on injection regimens, wide fluctuations in glucose levels, recurrent and significant hypoglycemic events, very young children requiring small amounts of insulin, or when lifestyle issues render an injection regimen especially difficult to manage. In short, virtually every youth with T1D has at least one of these indications. Consequently, caregivers should have an extensive conversation with both the child (if age appropriate) and family to explore the use an insulin pump.

It is essential that school-agers and adolescents themselves want to use an insulin pump. In fact, during the early days of pump therapy, word-of-mouth endorsements of insulin pumps at summer diabetes camps markedly increased the interest in the use of insulin pumps by youth with T1D being treated with insulin injections. The child and the adolescent should be shown the different types of insulin pumps, and an age-appropriate explanation on use of the pump should be provided so that the patient can make an informed decision. Our young patients need to understand that regardless of the type of pump they select, they will continuously have hardware attached to their body. Even if the parent desires the therapy, if the child is "forced" to use an insulin pump, the outcomes may not be as successful. Similarly, parents must agree with pursuing this therapy, as their support will be crucial to its success. Warning: families who miss a lot of diabetes care visits are not the best candidates for pump therapy.

The family also needs to have appropriate expectations for insulin pump therapy. They have to understand that the therapy is going to require significant effort on their part; perhaps even more than an insulin injection regimen. Moreover, using an insulin pump does not "cure" their diabetes, but it is a device to help them better manage their diabetes. Frequent glucose monitoring or use of a continuous glucose monitor is also important, and understanding carbohydrate counting is a necessity. They need to know how to manage illnesses with diabetes, the signs and symptoms of ketoacidosis, and when to call their diabetes provider for assistance.

Choosing an Insulin Pump

Currently in the United States, there are three main companies that make insulin pumps approved for use in pediatrics by the Federal Drug Administration (FDA). (Table 6.1). They are Insulet Corporation (Omnipod), Medtronic Diabetes (MiniMed 630G System and MiniMed 670G System), and Tandem Diabetes Care (t-slim X2 ™ Insulin Pump). The care provider needs to discuss the different options inherent with each pump in detail with the parents and patient (if appropriate). The first decision that a family needs to make is whether or not to have tubing. Many families will choose the Omnipod pump because of the ease of not having tubing, which is very appealing to many youth and their parents.

Table 6.1 Insulin pumps approved for pediatric use in the United States

Company	Pumps	Company contact
Insulet Corporation	Omnipod ®	https://www.myomnipod.com/Omnipod-system Phone: 1 800 591-3455
Medtronic	MiniMed™ 670G System MiniMed™ 630G System	https://www.medtronicdiabetes.com/home Phone: 1800 646-4633
Tandem® Diabetes Care	t:slim X2 ™ Insulin Pump	https://www.tandemdiabetes.com Phone: 1 877 801-6901

These pumps adhere well to the skin, but backup pod/supplies need to be available at all times for any pod problems.

If the family wants a pump with automation then both the Tandem t-slim X2 ™ and the Medtronic MiniMed 670G System should be shown to the family. If the child/adolescent is already wearing a DexCom G6 sensor, the Tandem t-slim X2™ may be chosen; whereas, those wearing the Guardian Connect CGM, the Medtronic MiniMed™ 670G System might be the pump of choice. In any event, the pros and cons of each pump system should be reviewed with the family so that an informed decision can be made.

Fulfilling the Promise of Insulin Pump Therapy

As noted in Chap. 5, no approach to insulin treatment of T1D is perfect without feedback control of insulin delivery based on real-time changes in sensor glucose levels. This is especially true during the overnight period, in which every night is an adventure. Einstein defined *insanity* as doing the same thing over and over again and always *expecting* a different result. In contrast, we define *insanity* for type 1 diabetes as using the same nighttime basal infusion doses over and over and always *getting* a different result. A major paradigm shift occurred with the introduction of commercially available real-time continuous glucose monitors (CGMs). While inaccurate readings, false alarms, and local irritation on the insertion site limited the use of early CGMs [7, 8], many of these obstacles have been overcome more recently. Indeed, at least some of the current generation CGMs are sufficiently accurate that they have replaced the need to use blood glucose meter testing to guide insulin therapy.

Of particular relevance to this chapter, the integration of current CGMs with insulin pumps has enabled information on sensor glucose levels to guide insulin dosing; namely, the holy grail of feedback control of insulin delivery based on real-time changes in sensor glucose levels. Nevertheless, fulfillment of the full potential of insulin pumps has been a relatively slow process. The earliest integrated CGM/pump systems involved a low-glucose suspend (LGS) feature that suspended insulin delivery when the CGM value reached a pre-set hypoglycemic level. Although the low glucose suspend feature significantly reduced the degree and duration of hypoglycemia, it did not prevent episodes of hypoglycemia events, particularly at night. In contrast, the predicted low glucose suspend (PLGS) device shuts off insulin delivery in advance of hypoglycemia, resulting in reductions in hypoglycemic events [9]. However, neither one of these advances helped to reduce the time patients spent in hyperglycemia.

The next step involved FDA approval of the Medtronic MiniMed 670G Hybrid Closed Loop system in 2016. In order to prevent overdelivery of insulin due to a system malfunction, this device requires users to count carbohydrates and to manually deliver the relatively large bolus doses of insulin for meals and snacks. On the other hand, the system varies insulin infusion rates between meals and during the overnight period based on feedback control of sensor glucose levels (Fig. 6.2). The safety and efficacy of this device was demonstrated in a pivotal clinical trial that involved both adults and adolescents with T1D [10, 11]. Additionally, the Tandem Control IQ Software, which also changes insulin delivery based on CGM imput (see Chap. 9), has been shown to improve glycemic control by decreasing the time spent in both hyperglycemia and hypoglycemia. A multitude of other automated insulin delivery systems are currently being investigated, including those with dual hormones, more advanced glucose sensor techniques, and more time in automated insulin delivery.

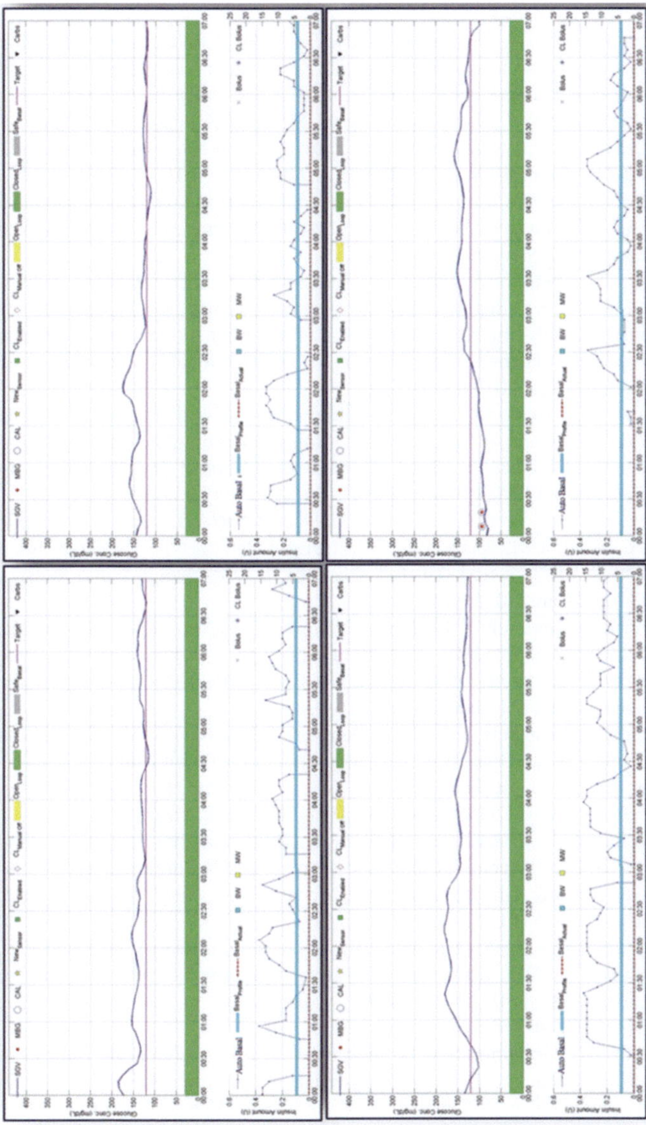

Fig. 6.2 Varying nighttime insulin delivery but always getting the same result the next morning

References

1. Tamborlane WV, Sherwin RS, Genel M, Felig P. Reduction to normal of plasma glucose in juvenile diabetics by subcutaneous administration of insulin with a portable infusion pump. N Engl J Med. 1979;300:573–8.
2. Tamborlane WV, Sherwin RS, Genel M, Felig P. Restoration of normal lipid and amino acid metabolism in diabetic patients treated with a portable insulin infusion pump. Lancet. 1979;1:1258–61.
3. Tamborlane WV, Sherwin RS, Genel M, Felig P. Outpatient management of juvenile-onset diabetics with a portable subcutaneous insulin infusion pump. Am J Med. 1980;68:190–6.
4. Grip ET, Svensson A, Miftaraj M, Eliasson B, Franzen S, Gudbjornsdottir S, Carlsson KS. Real world costs of continuous insulin pump therapy and multiple daily injections for type 1 diabetes: a population-based and propensity-matched cohort from the Swedish National Diabetes Registrar. Diabetes Care. 2019;42:545–52.
5. The DCCT Research Group. The effect of intensive diabetes treatment on the development and progression of long-term complications in insulin-dependent diabetes mellitus. The Diabetes Control and Complications Trial. N Engl J Med. 1993;329:977–86.
6. Miller KM, Foster NC, Beck RW, Bergenstal RM, Dubose S, DiMeglio LA, Maahs DM, Tamborlane WV. Current state of type 1 diabetes treatment in the US: updated data from the T1D exchange clinic registry. Diabetes Care. 2015;38:971–8.
7. Diabetes Research in Children Network (DirecNet) Study Group. The accuracy of the CGMS in children with type 1 diabetes: results of the Diabetes Research in Children Network (DirecNet) accuracy study. Diabetes Technol Ther. 2003;5:781–9.
8. Diabetes Research in Children Network (DirecNet) Study Group. The accuracy of the GlucoWatch G2 biographer in children with type 1 diabetes: results of the Diabetes Research in Children Network (DirecNet) accuracy study. Diabetes Technol Ther. 2003;5:791–800.
9. Forlenza GP, Buckingham BA, et al. Predicted low-glucose suspend reduces hypoglycemiain adults, adolescents and children with type 1 diabetes in an at-home randomized cross-over study. Diabetes Care. 2018;41:2155–61.
10. Bergenstal RM, Garg S, Weinzimer SA, Buckingham BA, Bode BW, Tamborlane WV, Kaufman FR. Safety of a hybrid closed-loop insulin delivery system in patients with type 1 diabetes. JAMA. 2016;316:1407–8.
11. Garg SK, Weinzimer SA, Tamborlane WV, Buckingham BA, Bode BW, Bailey TS, Brazg RL, Ilany J, Slover RH, Anderson SM, Bergenstal RM, Grosman B, Roy A, Cordero TL, Shin J, Lee SW, Kaufman FR. Glucose outcomes with the in-home use of a hybrid closed-loop insulin delivery system in adolescents and adults with type 1 diabetes. Diabetes Technol Ther. 2017;19:155–63.

7 Glucose Monitoring

William V. Tamborlane, Amy Steffen, and Michelle Van Name

Background

In the "really bad old days" of treating youth with type 1 diabetes (i.e., before 1980), we did not have a reliable method to monitor glycemic control. As illustrated in Fig. 7.1, the only tool that was available was measuring the concentration/amount of glucose in the urine. Of course, some of our families knew that regulating your insulin doses by the concentration of glucose in the urine was like trying to hit a baseball by its shadow (impossible). Another father reminded me that urine glucose was negative unless the blood sugar level was greater than 180 mg/dL. He said it was like trying to drive a car that only registered its speed at 180 miles/hour or greater.

We took it even further by having our families collect their child's urine during one of the weekend days over 4-time periods:

W. V. Tamborlane · A. Steffen · M. Van Name (✉)
Yale-New Haven Children's Hospital, Department of Pediatrics, Yale School of Medicine, New Haven, CT, USA
e-mail: William.tamborlane@yale.edu; amy.steffen@yale.edu; michelle.vanname@yale.edu

W. V. Tamborlane (ed.), *Diabetes in Children and Adolescents*, Contemporary Endocrinology, https://doi.org/10.1007/978-3-030-64133-7_7

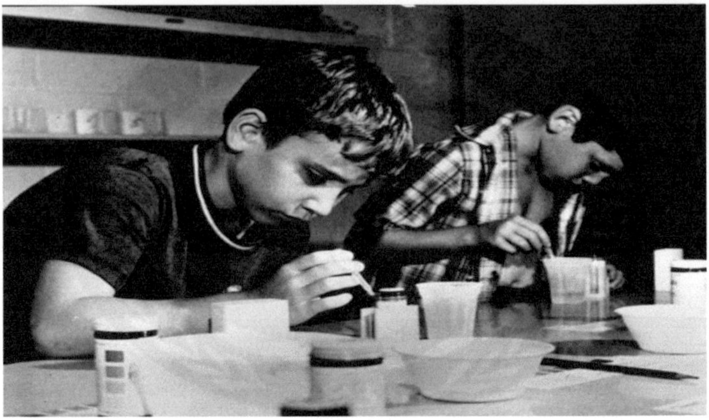

Fig. 7.1 Picture of youth with T1D checking urine glucose levels

breakfast to lunch, lunch to dinner, dinner to bedtime, and bedtime to breakfast. On the following Monday afternoon clinic session, parents would submit a list of the number of ounces of urine during each time period and bring in an aliquot of urine from each time interval to be tested for the glucose concentration by the hospital laboratory. As a postdoctoral fellow, I had to calculate the total amount of glucose in the urine in each time interval and, if the total amount of sugar was high during any time interval, we would make changes in the insulin dose. We actually thought that one day's data every 3 months was sufficient to adjust the treatment regimen. It is no wonder that youth in that era suffered many of the vascular complications of diabetes in relatively early adulthood.

Dawn of the Era of Intensive Treatment of Type 1 Diabetes (T1D)

It was not until the early 1980s when the treatment of T1D began to change for the better and advances in monitoring glycemic control were cornerstones.

Glycosylated Hemoglobin (HbA1c) It was well known that red blood cells of healthy individuals contained a small fraction of hemoglobin in which glucose was covalently bound. Glycosylated hemoglobin was also known as "fast hemoglobin" because it eluted from cation exchange resins more rapidly than non-glycosylated hemoglobin. A college friend who received a PhD in biochemistry told me that they would throw away blood samples with a lot of glucose attached to hemoglobin because they did not know what it meant. It was not until the end of the 1970s that investigators realized that the percent of covalently bound glycosylated hemoglobin in red blood cells was directly proportional to the average circulating blood sugar level in individuals with diabetes. It subsequently became apparent that measurements of glycosylated hemoglobin (AKA HbA1c) levels every 3 months provided a good approximation of overall glycemic control, since that was the average red cell turnover time for most individuals.

In simple terms, this meant that our youngsters could not just shape up their diabetes control during a day or two before clinic visits because prior poor glycemic control would show up in the HbA1c blood test. However, it was not until 1993 that the Diabetes Control and Complications Trial (DCCT) demonstrated that lowering HbA1c as close to normal as possible as early in the course of the disease as possible resulted in a marked delay in the development and progression of the microvascular complications of diabetes [1].

The good news was that HbA1c provided a simple surrogate marker for the risk of development of diabetes complications, namely, better control of blood glucose could delay or even prevent the development of vascular complications. The bad news was that HbA1c levels alone did not tell you how to achieve and maintain optimal glucose levels in individuals with diabetes.

Self-Blood Glucose Monitoring Coincidental to the introduction of glycosylated hemoglobin measurements, blood glucose meters were introduced that allowed patients themselves to measure blood glucose levels at home. A physician with T1D who I met when he was a resident in training, claims to have accidently stumbled on

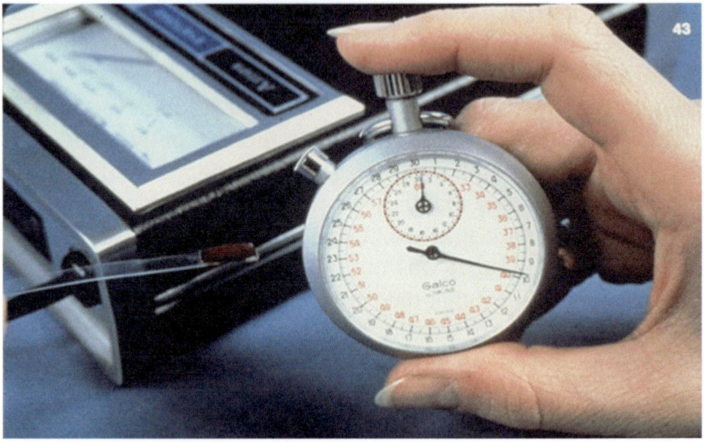

Fig. 7.2 First blood glucose meter

this idea when he worked in a medical laboratory prior to medical school that used the Ames Reflectance meter for rapid measurements of blood sugar levels (Fig. 7.2). This individual was confused about why he had sugar in his urine, even when he felt that his blood sugar level was low. To evaluate the discrepancy, he borrowed a Reflectance meter from the lab and demonstrated that his blood sugar level actually was low even when his urine tested positive for sugar. Long story short, blood glucose testing 3 or more times per day quickly gained popularity and blood glucose meters rapidly became more accurate, faster, and easier to use. An early landmark was the introduction of blood glucose meters that incorporated a memory function regarding the results, days, and times of previous tests. This improved reliability of blood glucose data beyond what was reported in the patient glucose diary [2].

Subsequently, blood glucose meter values could also be entered in the memory of mini-computers in advanced insulin pumps to calculate correction doses. To make it even easier, one company's pump started all blood glucose values at a default number of 100 mg/dL, which could then be moved up or down to equal the actual glucose level. I once asked a mother what her son's pre-meal blood glucose levels were like. She said, “that's easy, it's always 100 mg/dL—he never checks what his real blood glucose level is!”

Several generations of improvements of blood glucose meters over the past 40 years made self-monitoring of blood glucose (SMBG) central to the management of diabetes. It provided instant feedback, enabling the patient to make immediate adjustments if necessary. Moreover, tracking trends of change in blood glucose over the course of days or weeks supplied the patient and diabetes care provider with crucial information when adjusting insulin regimens or contemplating new therapeutic strategies. The newer glucose meters were very portable and required only a tiny drop of blood. As noted above, most had computerized memories to facilitate record keeping, a key feature in managing treatment of adolescents with diabetes. Nevertheless, SMBG measurements only provided brief snapshots of glucose levels before and occasionally 2–3 hours after meals and rarely during the night. It also became apparent that treatment of T1D would never be perfect until there was feedback control of insulin administration based on frequent, real-time measurements of changes in glucose concentrations.

Continuous Glucose Monitoring (CGM) The dawn of the new millennium saw the introduction of the first generation of CGM devices, namely, the Medtronic Continuous Glucose Monitoring System (CGMS) and the Gluco Watch Biographer [3, 4]. While these were important first steps, numerous studies highlighted the limitations of the first CGMs, which lead to their rapid disappearance from commercial sales. With further improvements in CGM devices, the JDRF CGM Study Group demonstrated that CGM could provide a better means to achieve optimal control of glucose than using blood glucose meter monitoring [5]. Of course, better glycemic control with CGM was only achieved in patients who used these early systems regularly, which represented a particularly great challenge for teenagers (Fig. 7.3). However, a more recent study reported more consistent use of CGM over time with the newest generation of CGM in adolescents and young adults with T1D [6].

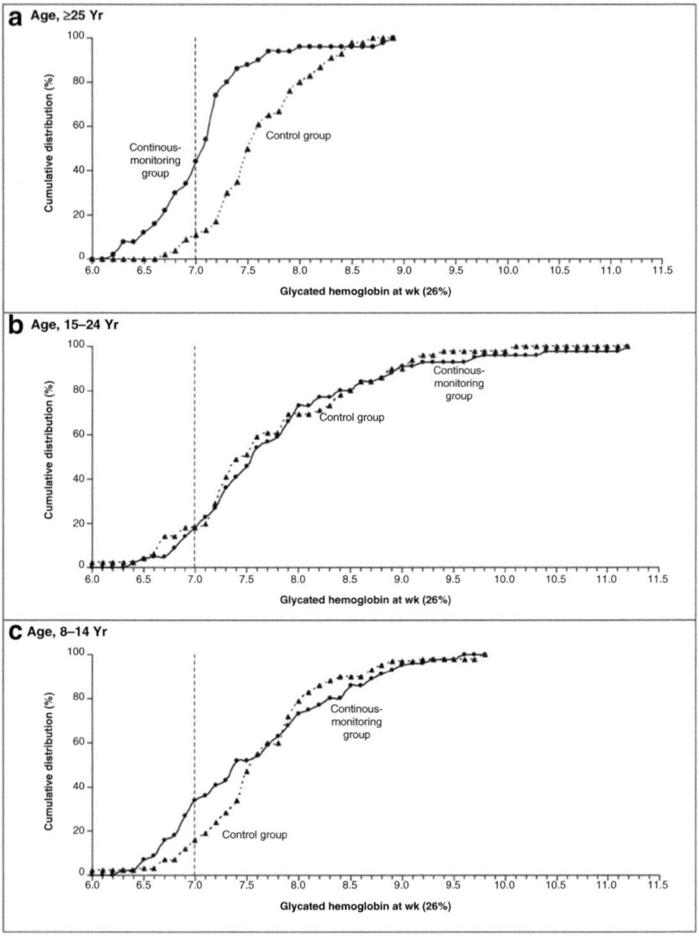

Fig. 7.3 Lowering HbA1c levels in T1D adults who wore CGM almost every day (Panel **a**). (From the The Juvenile Diabetes Research Foundation Continuous Glucose Monitoring Study Group [5] No difference in HbA1c was observed in 15-24 yr olds (Panel **b**) and 8-14 yr olds (Panell **c**). Copyright © (2008) Massachusetts Medical Society. Reprinted with permission)

The newest generation CGM sensors are inserted into the subcutaneous tissue. The electrochemical reaction between glucose oxidase in the sensor and interstitial glucose in the subcutaneous tissue produces an electric current that is directly proportional to the ambient glucose concentration that is read by the sensor and transmitted to a receiver.

CGM has become a critical tool in the management of diabetes in children and adolescents. Key features include accuracy, wear from 10 to 14 days, and use as replacement for fingerstick blood glucose monitoring. Additionally, sensor glucose trend arrows indicate the rate of glucose rise and fall, and some systems provide customizable alerts for high and low glucose thresholds. Web-based data-management software for real-time data upload to the cloud and real-time remote monitoring are features that are very attractive to parents of young children with T1D.

CGM in Very Young Children with T1D The SENCE Study Group recently evaluated the effects of CGM combined with family behavioral intervention (CGM+FBI) and CGM alone on glycemic outcomes and parental quality of life compared with blood glucose monitoring (BGM) in children age 2 to <8 years with type 1 diabetes [7]. It was a multicenter ($N = 14$), 6-month, randomized controlled trial that randomized 143 youth, age 2 to <8 years with type 1 diabetes. Primary analysis included treatment group comparisons of percent time in CGM ranges across follow-up visits. It is particularly noteworthy that ~90% of participants in the CGM groups used CGM ≥ 6 days/week over the 6 months of the study. Over the 6-month period, young children with T1D did not improve the time in target range (i.e., 70–180 mg/dL) but did significantly reduce time in hypoglycemia. The FBI also positively impacted parental well-being.

CGM Metrics In most current CGMs, the percentage of error is now <10%. Improved CGM accuracy has been accompanied by increased use of CGM in youth with T1D, and there is growing evidence that CGM use results in a significant HbA1c reductions in patients with T1D, whether patients are using insulin pump or multiple daily injection treatment. It is notable that many families in our practice with a child with new-onset T1D will initiate use of a CGM before consideration of starting insulin pump therapy, and many parents greatly appreciate the ability to monitor glucose levels in their child remotely through their cell phone. Of course, patients must use these devices regularly to obtain maximum benefit.

An added feature of regular use of current CGM devices has been the introduction of new metrics of glycemic control based on CGM profiles [8]. These include the following: (1) average daily glucose; (2) percentage of time in hypoglycemic ranges, i.e., <54 mg/dL and <70 mg/dL; (3) percentage of time in target range, i.e., 70–180 mg/dL; and (4) percentage of time in hyperglycemic range, i.e., ≥180 mg/dL and >250 mg/dL. CGM data can also be used to generate standardized reports with visual cues to determine glycemic patterns and to guide treatment decisions [8].

The ultimate goal is to integrate the current CGM devices with insulin pumps via a control algorithm that will enable automatic, feedback control of insulin delivery with little effort by the patient. Artificial pancreas projects have gained significant momentum for the past decade and are the topic of the next chapter.

References

1. The DCCT Research Group. The effect of intensive diabetes treatment on the development and progression of long-term complications in insulin-dependent diabetes mellitus. The Diabetes Cntrol and Complications Trial. N Engl J Med. 1993;329:977–86.
2. Mazze RS, Shamoon H, Pasmantier R, Lucido D, Murphy J, Hartmann K, Kuykendall V, Lopatin W. Reliability of blood glucose monitoring by patients with diabetes mellitus. Am J Med. 1984;77:211–7.
3. The Diabetes Research in Children Network (DirecNet) Study Group. The accuracy of the CGMS™ in children with type 1 diabetes: results of the Diabetes Research in Children Network (DirecNet) accuracy study. Diabetes Technol Ther. 2003;5:781–9.
4. The Diabetes Research in Children Network (DirecNet) Study Group. The accuracy of the GlucoWatch® G2™ biographer in children with type 1 diabetes: results of the Diabetes Research in Children Network (DirecNet) accuracy study. Diabetes Technol Ther. 2003;5:791–800.
5. JDRF CGM Study Group. Impact of continuous glucose monitoring in optimizing intensive treatment of type 1 diabetes in adults and children. N Engl J Med. 2008;359:1464–76.

6. Laffel LM, Kanapka LG, Beck RW, et al. Effect of continuous glucose monitoring ion adolescents and young adults. A randomized clinical trial. JAMA. 2020;323:2388–96.
7. Strategies to Enhance New CGM Use in Early Childhood (SENCE) Study Group. A randomized clinical trial assessing continuous glucose monitoring use with standardized education with or without a family behavioral intervention in very young children with type 1 diabetes. (in review).
8. Danne T, Nimri R, Battelino T, Bergenstal RM, Close KL, DeVries JH, Garg S, Heinemann L, Hirsch I, Amiel SA, Beck R, Bosi E, Buckingham B, Cobelli C, Dassau E, Doyle FJ 3rd, Heller S, Hovorka R, Jia W, Jones T, Kordonouri O, Kovatchev B, Kowalski A, Laffel L, Maahs D, Murphy HR, Nørgaard K, Parkin CG, Renard E, Saboo B, Scharf M, Tamborlane WV, Weinzimer SA, Phillip M. International consensus on use of continuous glucose monitoring. Diabetes Care. 2017;40:1631–40.

Automated Insulin Delivery

8

Stuart A. Weinzimer, Lori Carria, and Michelle Van Name

Background

In a relatively brief time span, we have seen a rapid evolution of advances in diabetes devices. For example, in the 15 years since the publication of the first studies of real-time CGM, there has been the rapid development of increasingly integrated pump/sensor systems with greater levels of automation and increased complexity of the automated algorithms required to run them. We have moved from simple systems that suspend insulin in response to a low glucose level, to hybrid closed-loop (HCL) systems that adjust between meal and overnight insulin delivery in real time to minimize both low and high glucose levels. Specifically, with HCL systems nighttime is no longer the worst time for individuals with T1D, since overnight insulin delivery varies automatically from one night to the next depending on real-time changes in sensor glucose levels. The specific aim is to prevent nocturnal hypoglycemia and to normalize fasting glucose levels each morning (Fig. 8.1).

S. A. Weinzimer (✉) · L. Carria · M. Van Name
Yale-New Haven Children's Hospital, Department of Pediatrics, Yale School of Medicine, New Haven, CT, USA
e-mail: stuart.weinzimer@yale.edu; lori.carria@yale.edu

W. V. Tamborlane (ed.), *Diabetes in Children and Adolescents*, Contemporary Endocrinology,
https://doi.org/10.1007/978-3-030-64133-7_8

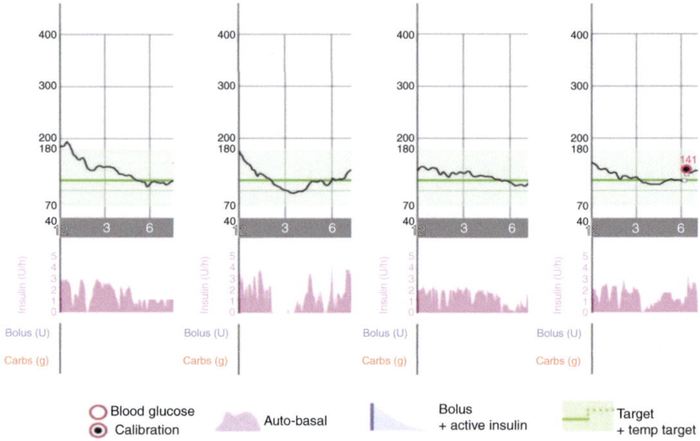

Fig. 8.1 Varying rates of overnight insulin infusion with automated HCL systems to achieve a consistent target of ~120 mg/dL every morning

Initial Small Steps in Automating Insulin Delivery

The first step in the development of automation and the simplest engineering algorithm was the threshold-suspend pump. As named, this system suspends basal insulin delivery when the glucose sensor records a reading below a predetermined hypoglycemic threshold at any given time of the day or night. Such a system has been likened to an automobile airbag; while not stopping hypoglycemia from occurring, it can minimize the damage by reducing the severity and duration of hypoglycemia. As demonstrated in a large-scale clinical trial conducted by Medtronic Diabetes, there was a 38% reduction in the time of exposure to hypoglycemia in participants using a threshold-suspend enabled sensor-augmented pump than a comparator sensor-augmented pump group without this feature [2]. By limiting the insulin pump suspension to 2 hours in duration, these systems did not increase the risk of significant hyperglycemia or ketosis, even if the pump should inappropriately suspend insulin delivery at normal or even high blood glucose levels [3]. Surprisingly, it took the FDA several years to approve the use of the first auto-suspend pump, even though most of the world recognized that it made no sense to continue to infuse insulin when blood glucose levels were low. The term for this is "clinical equipoise" or you do not have to do studies when you already know the answer!

The next incremental level of sophistication and improvement was the predictive low-glucose suspend system, which is designed to anticipate impending hypoglycemia before it actually occurs, based upon the trajectory of sensor glucose levels. These algorithms, which are available in several sensor-augmented pump systems, utilize linear regression of sensor glucose levels to predict the rate of fall of glucose and, if the threshold hypoglycemic level is expected to be reached within a given time horizon (e.g., 30 minutes), the basal insulin delivery will be suspended before the patient becomes hypoglycemic. Resumption of insulin delivery is based on the recovery of sensor glucose levels above a given threshold and a positive rate of change in sensor glucose levels. Several large-scale clinical trials have proven these systems effective in reducing exposure to hypoglycemia. For example, a randomized, 6-month parallel-group study showed that users of a predictive low-glucose suspend pump had an almost 50% reduction in time spent <63 mg/dL and <54 mg/dL compared to a sensor-augmented pump without this feature [4]. Similarly, a 6-week crossover study demonstrated a 31% reduction in glucose levels <70 mg/dL when the predictive suspend features were enabled [5]. It is important to note that clinically important reductions in hypoglycemia were achieved without an accompanying increase in hyperglycemia in both studies.

While suspend-on-low (threshold suspend) and suspend-before-low (predictive low-glucose suspend) systems are effective in reducing exposure to hypoglycemia, they do not automatically respond to hyperglycemia and are insufficient to lower A1c levels in the majority of patients struggling to meet strict glycemic targets. True "closed-loop" automated insulin delivery systems are defined by adjusting insulin delivery not only in response to actual or impending low glucose levels, but also high or rising glucose levels. More complex and sophisticated algorithms are required to effectively accomplish this task.

Multiple engineering approaches have been applied to the problem of glucose control, and while significant differences may be found among the various approaches, they all share the basic principle that the net rate of insulin delivery is determined by a combination of factors, including (1) the absolute glucose level; (2) the rate of rise or fall of the glucose level; (3) the timing and amount of previously administered insulin doses; and (4) conditions announced to the system (e.g., meals or exercise). Differences between the systems are primarily based on the mathematical models incorporated into their algorithms [6].

Current Hybrid Closed-Loop Systems

An important point that is common to any of the closed-loop systems currently available or approaching commercial release is that they are all "hybrid" closed-loop systems; namely, they require manual input of insulin at meal times. Hybrid closed-loop systems adjust basal insulin delivery in between meals and overnight, but users must deliver the appropriate amount of insulin for meals and snacks, based on the carbohydrate content of that meal, as well as whether the pre-meal glucose level is high or low. The original hybrid closed-loop concept involved manual administration of small, pre-meal priming doses of insulin to mitigate exaggerated post-prandial hyperglycemia due to delays in insulin absorption delivered automatically during the meal. For example, relying on a fully automated algorithm to detect the meal, based on the rising sensor glucose levels, results in a delay in insulin action that contributes to both early post-meal hyperglycemia and late post-meal hypoglycemia, only some of which can be corrected with algorithm modifications [7, 8]. The effectiveness of small, pre-meal priming doses of a rapid-acting insulin analog is shown in Fig. 8.2.

The HCL concept has changed over time in two major ways: (1) Current systems employ manual administration of large pre-meal doses of insulin to fully cover the carbohydrate content of the meal. The aim here is to mitigate the risk of over delivery of insulin due to a system malfunction by severely restricting the

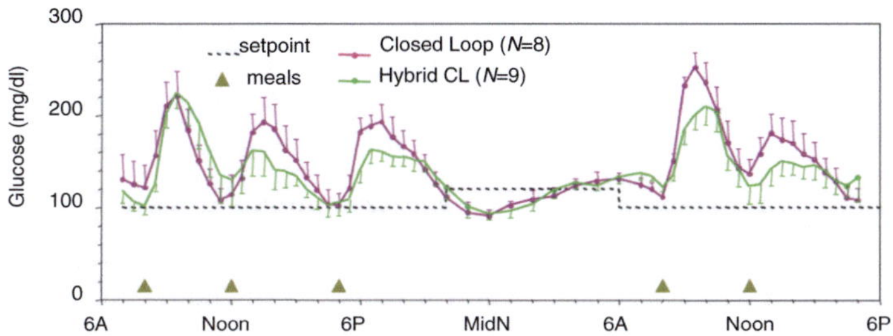

Fig. 8.2 Original hybrid closed-loop versus full closed-loop study. (Weinzimer S., et al. From Diabetes Care with permission)

amount of insulin that can be delivered automatically. (2) The system cleans up the back end by automatically adjusting basal insulin infusion rates after meals and during the night. Specifically, the sensor algorithm often completely suspends insulin delivery due to falling sensor glucose levels in the late, post-meal period.

The Medtronic 670G was first hybrid closed-loop system to become commercially available in the United States. In addition to requiring users to enter carbohydrate amounts and bolus manually at meal times, key features of this system include the following: (1) the sensor communicates glucose values directly to the pump, which houses the algorithm internally, without an intermediary controller/communicator device; (2) the algorithm has a fixed glucose target of 120 mg/dL, except when users choose an optional "impending exercise mode" set to 150 mg/dL; (3) the sensor requires calibration to a blood glucose meter value 2–3 times daily, or more frequently, as needed; and (4) the system has distinct "auto mode" and "manual mode" states. If all the required safety requirements are met, the system can operate in auto mode, in which the pump's closed-loop algorithm dynamically regulates between meal and overnight rates of insulin infusion; namely, there no longer is any fixed basal insulin infusion rates while the system is in auto mode. However, if any one of several safety signals occur, such as calibration issues with the sensor, extended time spent in hyperglycemia, or prolonged maximal insulin delivery rates, the system reverts to manual mode, returning the pump to the pre-set basal rates. Virtually, all of these features were intended to avoid automatic over delivery of insulin at all costs.

Clinical trials of the Medtronic 670G have demonstrated excellent safety and control results. In a single-cohort, longitudinal study in 124 adults and adolescents with T1D, mean A1c levels decreased from 7.4% at baseline to 6.9% after 3 months [9]. Time in glucose target, defined as time spent in 70–180 mg/dL range, increased significantly, from 60% to 69% in the adolescent cohort and from 67% to 74% in the adult cohort [10], with significant decreases in time spent in hyperglycemia and hypoglycemia. A subsequent single-arm 3-month study in children 7–13 years old showed similarly significant improvements from baseline to 3 months in A1c level (7.9–7.5%), time in target (56–65%), and reduced time spent in hyperglycemia and hypoglycemia [11].

The second system to become available in the United States is the Tandem t:slim X2 with Control-IQ Technology, which is also a hybrid closed-loop system, with the sensor sending glucose readings directly to the pump. However, there are important differences between this system and the Medtronic system, most notably in the sensor and toggling between auto and manual settings. The Tandem system incorporates the Dexcom G6 continuous glucose sensor, which does not require blood glucose entries or calibration and it allows users to "share" glucose values in real time remotely with designated caregivers. The Control-IQ algorithm utilizes not one, but several target glucose levels, depending on the time of day, and in addition to increasing basal insulin delivery for hyperglycemia, the system can also deliver automatic correction boluses, if the basal adjustments are insufficient to normalize glucose levels.

Clinical trials of the Tandem Control-IQ system have demonstrated similar levels of achieved time in target and HbA1c levels as in the Medtronic 670G trials. However, the Tandem Control-IQ studies have been randomized controlled trials with an open-loop control arm and a longer duration of treatment, making these studies considerably more robust. A multi-center study of 168 participants age 14–71, randomized in 2:1 manner to hybrid-closed loop control versus senor-augmented pump therapy, demonstrated an improvement in time in range in the closed-loop group from 61%

at baseline to 71% at 6 months, while in the control group the time in range was unchanged. The closed-loop group also saw concomitant reductions in time in hyperglycemia. Mean baseline-adjusted difference in HbA1c levels at the end of the study was 0.33% in favor of the closed-loop group. Most impressively, subjects in this trial were able to stay in closed-loop mode over 90% of the time, a key indicator of ease of use of the system.

A third hybrid closed-loop system, developed by Insulet, is currently in clinical trials. This device will differ from the Medtronic and Tandem systems in that as an "untethered" patch pump, the system is controlled through a smartphone device, which relays communications between the glucose sensor (in this case, the Dexcom G6), and the "pod." Early phase, semi-ambulatory studies have demonstrated feasibility of this system [12], and a large-scale pivotal trial is ongoing at the time of this writing.

Future Automated Insulin Delivery Systems

The field of automated insulin delivery is continuing to evolve rapidly. The "next generation" of systems has already begun to address the need for manual meal boluses and the addition of additional hormones. Dual-hormone systems comprising both insulin and glucagon are particularly attractive in their potential to reduce the risk of hypoglycemia even under the challenging conditions of exercise. Short-duration studies have shown promising results in the improvement in time in range, as well as a reduction in hypoglycemia and need for carbohydrate rescue [13]. Dual-hormone systems have been limited by requirements to reconstitute the glucagon daily for use in the pump, but new glucagon preparations have been approved that have long-term stability in liquid form and do not require reconstitution for use. Other hormones, such as pramlintide, which function within a closed-loop system to reduce post-prandial glycemic excursions by attenuating inappropriate meal-related endogenous glucagon secretion, have shown preliminary effectiveness but require further study [14–16]. Sodium-glucose transporter inhibitors (SGLTI), which mitigate post-prandial hyperglycemia in an insulin-independent manner by increasing renal clearance, have also generated excitement as an adjunctive agent to insulin in closed-loop systems although concerns remain about their safety.

The full capabilities of automated control systems have yet to be explored. Most recently, there has been considerable interest in incorporating other inputs to the control algorithms beyond just the glucose levels. Additional functionalities such as heart rate monitors or accelerometers may enable these systems to detect when a wearer is exercising and adjust the insulin delivery algorithms automatically to account for changing insulin requirements. The incorporation of global positioning systems and their integration with user calendars and machine learning algorithms may even enable a closed-loop system to detect when a wearer is driving to his or her weekly spinning class and adjust the insulin delivery algorithms before the exercise even starts. We have been testing systems that will allow wearers to use their own smartphones as controller devices, obviating the need for separate controller devices, and enabling customizable alerts and alarms as well as dynamically assigning "sharing" roles to multiple care providers/allies based on time of day or other individual preference [17].

Despite the increasing power and complexity of these systems, or perhaps because of this, it is becoming increasingly well recognized that the ultimate success of automated insulin delivery will depend not only on designing the best pump, sensor, or algorithm, but also on understanding the human factors involved in how people will use these systems. Our initial look into these issues taught us that people approach automation with varying levels of trust and expectations; it is clear that the process of educating users about these systems must begin before they are even prescribed. People must understand not only what the systems are capable (and incapable) of achieving, the level of engagement that must be maintained in order to successfully operate these devices, and even understand their own feelings about relinquishing daily decision-making about insulin doses over to a machine [18, 19]. As we are learning more about the initiation and maintenance of hybrid closed-loop systems in people with diabetes, structured education and training programs are also beginning to be developed and evaluated [20, 21]. A comprehensive and standardized approach will help ensure that as the pool of users and trainers expand over time, content will be delivered effectively and follow-up care optimized. This process will continue to evolve as new systems and technologies enter the market, but the overall importance of education on the success of the implementation of technology cannot be overestimated.

As the automation and integration of advanced diabetes devices continues to advance rapidly, accelerating the development and testing of new devices at an ever-increasing pace, we are optimistic that they will realize the dream of improving glycemic control and reducing the burden for those living with T1D.

References

1. Foster NC, Beck RW, Miller KM, et al. State of type 1 diabetes management and outcomes from the T1D exchange in 2016-2018. Diabetes Technol Ther. 2019;21(2):66–72. https://doi.org/10.1089/dia.2018.0384.
2. Bergenstal RM, Klonoff DC, Garg SK, et al. Threshold-based insulin-pump interruption for reduction of hypoglycemia. N Engl J Med. 2013;369(3):224–32. https://doi.org/10.1056/NEJMoa1303576.
3. Sherr JL, Palau Collazo M, Cengiz E, et al. Safety of nighttime 2-hour suspension of Basal insulin in pump-treated type 1 diabetes even in the absence of low glucose. Diabetes Care. 2014;37(3):773–9. https://doi.org/10.2337/dc13-1608.
4. Abraham MB, Nicholas JA, Smith GJ, et al. Reduction in hypoglycemia with the Predictive Low-Glucose Management System: a long-term randomized controlled trial in adolescents with type 1 diabetes. Diabetes Care. 2018;41(2):303–10. https://doi.org/10.2337/dc17-1604.
5. Forlenza GP, Li Z, Buckingham BA, et al. Predictive Low-Glucose Suspend reduces hypoglycemia in adults, adolescents, and children with type 1 diabetes in an at-home randomized crossover study: results of the PROLOG trial. Diabetes Care. 2018;41(10):2155–61. https://doi.org/10.2337/dc18-0771.
6. Doyle FJ 3rd, Huyett LM, Lee JB, Zisser HC, Dassau E. Closed-loop artificial pancreas systems: engineering the algorithms. Diabetes Care. 2014;37(5):1191–7. https://doi.org/10.2337/dc13-2108.
7. Weinzimer SA, Steil GM, Swan KL, Dziura J, Kurtz N, Tamborlane WV. Fully automated closed-loop insulin delivery versus semiautomated hybrid control in pediatric patients with type 1 diabetes using an artificial

pancreas. Diabetes Care. 2008;31(5):934–9. https://doi.org/10.2337/dc07-1967.
8. Ruiz JL, Sherr JL, Cengiz E, et al. Effect of insulin feedback on closed-loop glucose control: a crossover study. J Diabetes Sci Technol. 2012;6(5):1123–1130. Published 2012 Sep 1. https://doi.org/10.1177/193229681200600517.
9. Bergenstal RM, Garg S, Weinzimer SA, et al. Safety of a hybrid closed-loop insulin delivery system in patients with type 1 diabetes. JAMA. 2016;316(13):1407–8. https://doi.org/10.1001/jama.2016.11708.
10. Garg SK, Weinzimer SA, Tamborlane WV, et al. Glucose outcomes with the in-home use of a hybrid closed-loop insulin delivery system in adolescents and adults with type 1 diabetes. Diabetes Technol Ther. 2017;19(3):155–63. https://doi.org/10.1089/dia.2016.0421.
11. Forlenza GP, Pinhas-Hamiel O, Liljenquist DR, et al. Safety evaluation of the MiniMed 670G system in children 7-13 years of age with type 1 diabetes. Diabetes Technol Ther. 2019;21(1):11–9. https://doi.org/10.1089/dia.2018.0264.
12. Sherr JL, Buckingham BA, Forlenza GP, et al. Safety and performance of the Omnipod hybrid closed-loop system in adults, adolescents, and children with type 1 diabetes over 5 days under free-living conditions. Diabetes Technol Ther. 2020;22(3):174–84. https://doi.org/10.1089/dia.2019.0286.
13. El-Khatib FH, Balliro C, Hillard MA, et al. Home use of a bihormonal bionic pancreas versus insulin pump therapy in adults with type 1 diabetes: a multicentre randomised crossover trial [published correction appears in Lancet. 2017 Jan 28;389(10067):368] [published correction appears in Lancet. 2017 Feb 4;389(10068):e2]. Lancet. 2017;389(10067):369–80. https://doi.org/10.1016/S0140-6736(16)32567-3.
14. Weinzimer SA, Sherr JL, Cengiz E, et al. Effect of pramlintide on prandial glycemic excursions during closed-loop control in adolescents and young adults with type 1 diabetes. Diabetes Care. 2012;35(10):1994–9. https://doi.org/10.2337/dc12-0330.
15. Sherr JL, Patel NS, Michaud CI, et al. Mitigating meal-related glycemic excursions in an insulin-sparing manner during closed-loop insulin delivery: the beneficial effects of adjunctive Pramlintide and Liraglutide. Diabetes Care. 2016;39(7):1127–34. https://doi.org/10.2337/dc16-0089.
16. Haidar A, Tsoukas MA, Bernier-Twardy S, et al. A novel dual-hormone insulin-and-pramlintide artificial pancreas for type 1 diabetes: a randomized controlled crossover trial. Diabetes Care. 2020;43(3):597–606. https://doi.org/10.2337/dc19-1922.
17. Deshpande S, Pinsker JE, Zavitsanou S, et al. Design and clinical evaluation of the Interoperable Artificial Pancreas System (iAPS) smartphone app: interoperable components with modular design for progressive arti-

ficial pancreas research and development. Diabetes Technol Ther. 2019;21(1):35–43. https://doi.org/10.1089/dia.2018.0278.
18. Iturralde E, Tanenbaum ML, Hanes SJ, et al. Expectations and attitudes of individuals with type 1 diabetes after using a hybrid closed loop system. Diabetes Educ. 2017;43(2):223–32. https://doi.org/10.1177/0145721717697244.
19. Tanenbaum ML, Iturralde E, Hanes SJ, et al. Trust in hybrid closed loop among people with diabetes: perspectives of experienced system users. J Health Psychol. 2020;25(4):429–38. https://doi.org/10.1177/1359105317718615.
20. Messer LH, Forlenza GP, Wadwa RP, et al. The dawn of automated insulin delivery: a new clinical framework to conceptualize insulin administration. Pediatr Diabetes. 2018;19(1):14–7. https://doi.org/10.1111/pedi.12535.
21. Messer LH, Berget C, Forlenza GP. A clinical guide to advanced diabetes devices and closed-loop systems using the CARES paradigm. Diabetes Technol Ther. 2019;21:462.

Medical Nutritional Therapy

9

Paulina Rose, Mary Savoye,
and Eileen Tichy

Background

Type 1 diabetes (T1D) is an autoimmune disorder due to severely reduced or absolute deficiency of endogenous insulin secretion. Historically, people diagnosed with diabetes in the early 1900s and prior to the discovery of insulin were prescribed the Allan Starvation Diet that was severely restricted in carbohydrate intake and consisted of fat, protein, limited amounts of non-starchy vegetables, and daily exercise. After the discovery of insulin, the diet prescription became more relaxed, but it was still low in carbohydrates (<20%), high in fat (>70%), moderate in protein (<10%), and absent of concentrated sugars [7]. It is noteworthy that youth with T1D were encouraged to avoid simple sugars well into the 1980s. At that time, grandparents could be heard to admonish their grandchildren with T1D by saying, "No more sweets or cookies for you." Conversely, one of our adult patients enrolled in the DCCT recalled having to remind her mother when she was a

P. Rose (✉) · M. Savoye · E. Tichy
Yale-New Haven Children's Hospital, Department of Pediatrics,
Yale School of Medicine, New Haven, CT, USA
e-mail: paulina.rose@yale.edu

W. V. Tamborlane (ed.), *Diabetes in Children and Adolescents*, Contemporary Endocrinology,
https://doi.org/10.1007/978-3-030-64133-7_9

teenager that she could not eat her birthday cake because she had diabetes. At another clinic visit, one of our mothers complained about two things: (1) her daughter with T1D was getting hypoglycemic before lunch and (2) Mom was finding candy wrappers under her daughter's bed. We took care of both problems by prescribing a candy bar every morning at 10 AM. On the return visit, Mom complained that her son wanted to know why he could not have a 10 AM candy bar at school, even though he did not have diabetes!

With the advent of new insulin formulations and advances in diabetes technology, flexibility in meal planning resulted, carbohydrate intake increased, and the goal of the dietary prescription became individualization, chiefly to adapt insulin therapy to the nutritional needs and lifestyle of the person. Despite advances in therapy, dietary management of diabetes remains one of the most challenging aspects of treatment and a key to diabetes control.

Medical Nutritional Therapy

Current guidelines for healthy eating for youth with T1D are the same as for children without diabetes. The main difference being that children with T1D must take insulin. The ISPAD guidelines of 2014 specify that the goal of a proper diet is to provide sufficient energy for appropriate growth and weight maintenance, to ameliorate long-term complications, and to prevent acute complications such as severe hypoglycemia and diabetic ketoacidosis [1]. Energy intake should be distributed as 45–55% carbohydrate with less than 10% added sugars, 10–20% protein, and 30–35% fat. Saturated fat should be limited to <10% and polyunsaturated, monounsaturated, and Omega 3s fatty acids should be encouraged [7].

Recently, these dietary recommendations have been challenged as some studies have shown that lower carbohydrate intake results in reduced post-prandial hyperglycemia while other observational studies have reported lower HbA1c levels associated with a lower carbohydrate intake [1, 2, 19]. However, there is general agreement that carbohydrates should not be restricted in children and adolescents with T1D, as it may adversely affect growth and development. Moreover, very low-carbohydrate diets restrict or eliminate many foods that are important sources of micronutrients; therefore, dietary recommendations must be individualized and be flexible rather than rigid and dogmatic [3].

A balanced diet that emphasizes nutrient-dense foods is recommended for the entire family, not only for the child with diabetes. Families should be educated on macronutrient composition of the diet; the effects of macronutrients on blood glucose; carbohydrate counting or estimation; hypoglycemia treatment and prevention; timing of insulin action and meals; handling special or festive occasions; weight management; and prevention of disordered eating. Additionally, barriers to healthy eating should be addressed during nutrition education, including parent's perception that healthy eating is costlier, more time is spent preparing healthy meals, concerns related to social influences on eating, and feelings that their child with T1D might be seen as different [6]. Nutritional advice should also take into consideration cultural, ethnic, and family traditions [17]. It is important that the whole family be involved in making dietary changes based on healthy eating. It is also noteworthy that youth with T1D are no longer "thin." In fact, approximately 36–39% of youth with T1D have BMI z-scores in the overweight to obese ranges.

The type of insulin regimen prescribed will determine the nutrition care plan or vice versa; mainly, carbohydrate intake and insulin should be balanced against each other. Fixed doses of insulin will require that a meal plan with fixed carbohydrate intake be established and maintained consistently from day to day. The exception to this rule is during the honeymoon phase of T1D. During that period, residual endogenous insulin secretion can often make up for modest increases in carbohydrate intake.

Injections of rapid-acting insulin analogs before meals in combination with long-acting insulin analogs to cover the overnight period or use of an insulin pump, allow for more flexibility in food intake as insulin doses are matched to the planned carbohydrate intake for each meal (AKA basal-bolus therapy). As mentioned in Chap. 4, we initially treat patients with a standard intake of carbohydrate for each main meal, so that we will be better able to establish the insulin to carbohydrate ratio. Subsequently, patients and caregivers will be able to calculate pre-meal insulin doses based on the amount of carbohydrate to be consumed with each meal. The latter approach of adjusting insulin doses based on variations in appetite works best in the long run.

Carbohydrates

This is the macronutrient that impacts blood glucose the most. The amount of carbohydrate consumed and the amount and timing of insulin injections are the main factors that determine the rise in plasma glucose after meals. Carbohydrates are composed of chains of glucose molecules that are broken down during digestion by enzymes (saliva and pancreatic enzymes). They pass from the stomach into the small intestine from whence they are absorbed into the bloodstream. The primary role of carbohydrates is to provide energy to the cells in the body [4]. The classification of types of carbohydrates is shown in Table 9.1.

Carbohydrates can only be absorbed in the bloodstream in the form of mono-saccharides. Fiber is not digested nor absorbed and passes out of the body. The liver stores glucose in the form of glycogen, which consists of long chains of glucose molecules.

Table 9.1 Types of carbohydrates

Sugars (digestible)	
Mono-saccharides	Glucose, fructose (fruit sugar), galactose (milk sugar)
Di-saccharides	Sucrose (table sugar), lactose (milk sugar), maltose (malt sugar)
Polyols	Sugar alcohols: sorbitol. Mannitol, xylitol
Starches (digestible)	
Amylose	Chains of glucose molecules in starchy vegetables
Amylopectin	Chains of glucose molecules found in breads, cereals, and grains
Fiber (not digestible)	Cellulose, hemi-cellulose, pectin, gums, mucilage, fructans

The terms "complex carbohydrate" and "simple sugars" are no longer used. There are naturally occurring sugars in the cell walls of plants (fructose) and in milk (lactose) and sugars that are added during food processing found in beverages, cookies, cakes, candy, desserts, cereals, flavored yogurts, condiments, and prepared foods. The Nutrition Facts label does not always distinguish between naturally occurring sugars and added sugars. Foods with excessive amounts of added sugars tend to be energy dense and nutritionally deficient. Traditionally, foods with added sucrose have been restricted in people with diabetes, but studies have shown that an equal amount of sucrose or starch in a meal affects the plasma glucose rise similarly [7]. Nevertheless, the USDA recommends consuming a healthy diet that limits sugar intake to <10% of total calories [15]. Giving emphasis to healthy carbohydrates before consuming concentrated sugar is a reasonable approach that allows children with diabetes to partake in the occasional sweet treat, especially during consumption of mixed meals that include fat, which slows gastric emptying.

Foods that contain carbohydrate include the following:

- Breads, cereals, grains.
- Pasta, rice, beans, and legumes.
- Starchy vegetables such as potatoes, winter squash, corn, and peas.
- Fruit and fruit juices.
- Dairy products such as milk and yogurt. Even though cheese is made from milk, it does not contain carbohydrates. Fresh cheese such as cottage cheese and farmer's cheese have a small amount of carbohydrate.
- Chocolate, cookies, candy, sugar, soft drinks, and other sweetened beverages.

Healthy carbohydrates are foods that are minimally processed such as unrefined grains, beans and legumes, whole fruits, vegetables, and dairy products. These are excellent sources of micronutrients and phytochemicals and have a lower glycemic index;

some of these foods are also high in fiber. The diet should emphasize these types of carbohydrates above their refined counterparts. Intrinsic fiber present in unrefined plant foods may help slow down the post-prandial rise in plasma glucose [13].

Two types of fiber are present in foods, soluble and insoluble. Soluble fiber, such as found in barley, oats, legumes, ground flax seeds, chia seeds, apples, citrus, and berries, is believed to slow digestion and absorption of nutrients because it forms a viscous gel in the digestive tract that holds water and binds glucose. It also traps and excretes bile acids and may reduce total cholesterol and LDL concentrations [13]. Additionally, it provides fuel for friendly bacteria, improving the gut microbiome. Insoluble fiber creates bulk in the intestinal fecal matter and promotes regularity. Both types of fiber alleviate constipation. Foods are stripped of their natural fiber during processing, and sadly, the standard American diet, which is high in animal protein, fat, sugar, and refined starch, is very low in fiber.

It has been observed in a series of reviews and meta-analysis that people with the highest consumption of dietary fiber in comparison to the lowest consumption have a 15–30% reduction in all-cause mortality [5]. Fruits and vegetables are good sources of fiber, but children with and without T1D eat on average fewer than the recommended intake of five servings per day. Switching to unrefined whole grain bread, choosing cereals with fiber, and offering vegetables with meals and fruits with snacks can increase fiber intake.

Sweeteners There are nutritive sweeteners and non-nutritive sweeteners or artificial sugars. Some manufacturers market food products as "no sugar added" which can be misleading. The food may not have extra added sugar, but it still contains intrinsic sugar. A prime example is frozen fruit juice bars or applesauce.

Sucrose, commonly known as table sugar, used to be restricted for people with diabetes. However, as noted previously, an equal amount of sugar or starch in a meal can have similar increases in plasma glucose after a meal. Consequently, children with T1D can enjoy an occasional treat that contains sugar. If the portions of other carbohydrates in the meal are reduced and replaced with sugar, a consistent carbohydrate target can be maintained. In addition, more rapid-acting insulin can be given to compensate for the increased amount of carbohydrate. Foods high in sugar have low nutritional profiles and are high in calories, which can contribute to excessive weight gain if consumed too often. Thus, sweets should be incorporated as the occasional treat rather than the norm.

Fructose has a low glycemic index, which suggests it could be a good choice for people with T1D. It does not affect plasma glucose directly; it is transformed to glucose in the liver and can have harmful effects on plasma lipids and cause weight gain. Many food products in the United States are sweetened with high fructose corn syrup, which has been implicated in the increasing rates of obesity and non-alcoholic fatty liver disease or NAFLD [14]. Both sucrose and fructose yield 4 calories/gram.

Sugar-alcohols, also called polyols, are used by food manufacturers to lower the carbohydrate content of foods; that is, they are often used in "sugar-free" candy, ice cream, and pastry. The names end in "ol" (e.g., sorbitol). The energy yield is about 2 calories/gram of sugar alcohol. It is recommended when counting carbohydrates that half the grams of sugar alcohol be subtracted from the total grams of carbohydrates. Large amounts of sorbitol can cause intestinal discomfort and diarrhea in some people.

Non-nutritive sweeteners contain zero or few calories and are available in the United States as Acesulfame K (Sweet One), Aspartame (Nutra-Sweet, Equal), Saccharin (Sweet'n Low), and Sucralose (Splenda). They are found in many food products labeled "diet." Food manufacturers use the term "low sugar" when the amount of sugar in the original food is reduced and blended with an artificial sugar. Some of these sweeteners have a bad reputation that is mostly anecdotal. The FDA approves all sweeteners and determines a safe daily intake that includes a 100-fold safety factor, which greatly exceeds average consumption [6]. They are approved for people with diabetes in moderation, including children and pregnant women. Recently, novel sweeteners have come into market such as Stevia, Monk fruit, and Allulose. They are extracted from plants and considered by some as "more natural" and safer. They taste sweeter than sugar and contain no calories. However, they can have an unpleasant aftertaste, which some people dislike.

Glycemic Index (GI)

This refers to the effect of various carbohydrate foods on plasma glucose level in comparison to glucose alone. Typically, rate and magnitude of the rise in plasma glucose following ingestion of 50 grams of a carbohydrate containing food is compared to 50 grams of glucose or white bread. Glucose has a glycemic index of 100, and other foods are ranked against it. Specifically, carbohydrates are classified as having a glycemic index that is:

- Low: <55
- Medium: 55–<70
- High: >70

However, there is much variability within each food category and between and within persons as many characteristics affect the glycemic response such as particle size, fiber content, ripeness, food preparation, degree of processing, acidity, and other factors related to food ingestion and digestion [10]. Because of the complexity of this, the American Diabetes Association does not recommend the use of GI as a primary dietary tool for glucose control [7]. Of note, the GI of a food affects post-prandial glycemia, not fasting glycemia.

Substituting high GI foods with low GI foods may slightly lower the glucose spike that occurs after eating. This has been shown to lower HbA1c by ~0.5% in some studies but not others [10]. Foods with medium to low GI appear to cause a blunted rise on blood glucose and may modestly improve glycemic control [16]. The insulin bolus can be increased judiciously to counteract the spike of high GI foods, but beware of the potential risk for hypoglycemia in the late post-meal period.

Persons with T1D can learn to recognize their own responses to different foods and develop strategies to adjust meal-related insulin accordingly. One approach is to select mostly foods with a low or medium GI value. When consuming high GI foods, it would be beneficial to balance them in the same meal with low GI foods. High GI foods can be selected in instances when the glucose needs to be raised rather quickly such as pre-exercise.

The timing of the insulin bolus in relation to the meal can be a useful tool to optimize post-prandial control [2]. Specifically, giving insulin 15 to 20 minutes prior to eating can help blunt the spike. Due to the delayed action of subcutaneous insulin, it is recommended to give the bolus prior to eating rather than giving it after or during the meal, but exceptions can be made for toddlers and other children with unpredictable appetites. Insulin pumps have the advantage of splitting the bolus into multiple parts; for example, half upfront and the rest after the meal is finished. Improving dietary quality and mealtime routines through nutrition education also can help improve post-prandial hyperglycemia, not just insulin adjustment.

Protein

This macronutrient is found mostly in animal products, although there are sources of vegetarian protein in combination with carbohydrates. Protein is found in meat, poultry, pork, fish and seafood, eggs, cheese and dairy products, nuts and seeds, beans/legumes, and grains. Pure protein is made up of amino acids. In non-diabetic individuals, meals with a mixture of carbohydrates and protein usually do not stimulate the secretion of glucagon in the pancreas. However, in patients with T1D, protein stimulates the release of glucagon even in meals that are high in carbohydrate. Acute, meal-stimulated secretion of glucagon, in turn, stimulates glucose production by the liver, which contributes to post-meal hyperglycemia.

The addition of protein to a snack does not prevent hypoglycemia, but it contributes to satiety. Young children tend not to eat sufficient protein to stimulate an increase in plasma glucose, but adolescents and young adults often do. The RDA for protein for children varies from 1.5 grams/kg/day for infants to 0.85 grams/kg/day for adolescent males through age 18 years. This corresponds to 10–15% of calories from protein. Some adolescents interested in weight training may start taking protein supplements to build extra muscle on the advice of their coaches. Care must be taken to discuss a safe amount of protein supplements that do not interfere with kidney function.

Paterson et al. [18] looked at the effect of protein alone and found that a moderate amount of <50 grams did not affect glycemia. However, 75–100 grams of protein in the absence of carbohydrate and fat significantly increased glucose similarly to 20 grams of carbohydrate without insulin [18]. Calculating insulin requirements for a standard meal is usually based on the grams of carbohydrate, but larger amounts of protein in that meal may need a few additional units of insulin. If using an insulin pump, an extended or dual wave bolus can be programmed to prevent late, post-meal hyperglycemia. In time, trial and error and BG excursions will reveal the appropriate approach for each individual.

Fat

Many individuals falsely believe that dietary fat increases blood glucose directly, but this is not the case. In fact, just the opposite is true: fat slows the emptying of the stomach and consequently, the absorption of glucose. Fat causes a delay in glucose rise, which can last several hours, dependent on the amount of fat in the meal. We demonstrated this many years ago with pizza, which caused a prolonged increase in glucose after a high fat pizza meal.

Saturated fats and trans-fatty acids are atherogenic, namely, implicated in the development of arteriosclerosis and heart disease, which are common, long-term comorbidities that have their origin in youth with T1D. Fat comes in solid and liquid form. Saturated fats are solid at room temperature. These are found in red meats, pork products, dairy products, butter, palm oil, and coconut oil. Liquid fats are oils, classified as poly-unsaturated and mono-unsaturated. Mono-unsaturated fats such as olive oil, rapeseed oil, nut oils, and avocados are heart-healthy and should be consumed more than the others. Omega-3 fatty acids are found in fatty fish, walnuts, and flax seeds. They are also cardio-protective and in large doses may lower triglyceride levels. People in general should consume 2–3 servings per week of foods high in Omega-3s.

Trans-fats should be avoided or limited. These are liquid oils that have been hydrogenated through a chemical process and turned into solid fats. They are added to many snack foods to prolong shelf life, such as cookies, commercial bakery products, chips, and chocolate and are listed in the ingredients as "partially hydrogenated vegetable oil" or "vegetable shortening." They are being phased out of the food system gradually but beware if the replacement is "palm oil" which is highly saturated. Fats are calorically dense, providing 9 calories/gram.

Carbohydrate Counting

This meal planning method can improve metabolic control without causing an increase in weight and insulin requirements [8]. It is recommended for children using fixed doses of insulin as well as those using basal-bolus therapy by multiple daily insulin injections or insulin pumps. There are different ways of estimating carbohydrate content of meals, some are simple and some more advanced. The total carbohydrate content of a meal is more important when determining the amount of insulin units required than the type of the carbohydrate [7]. Nonetheless, the quality of carbohydrates also affects the glycemic response and should not be ignored.

Carbohydrate content of foods can be found using the Nutrition Facts panel on processed foods or published databases with nutritional information. Caregivers need to pay careful attention to the portion sizes in food labels. Carbohydrates are measured in the number of grams or as carbohydrate exchanges. Each exchange is a serving of starch, fruit, or milk that has 15 grams of carbohydrate on average. Free foods or low-carbohydrate foods have fewer than 5 grams of carbohydrate. A serving of meat (1 oz) contains no carbohydrates. A serving of fat (5 grams) has no carbohydrates but contains many calories. Protein and fat content, while important to an overall healthy meal plan, are not counted as a general rule. However, they can impact the absorption of carbohydrates. The exchange lists can facilitate estimation of carbohydrate content of meals for persons with low numeracy skills and is appropriate when using fixed insulin doses.

Counting Carbohydrates All packaged foods have a Nutrition Facts panel. Before a meal or snack, the youth or caregiver should use a measuring cup or spoon or weigh on a scale the amount of food desired and compare it to the serving size listed on the food label. The label lists the total carbohydrate grams per serving—the sugar grams are ignored because they are included in the total grams of carbohydrate. The fiber grams should be deducted from the total grams when they approximate 5 grams of fiber or more. Likewise, if the label lists sugar alcohols such as sorbitol, xylitol, or mannitol, half of the polyol grams should be subtracted from the total grams of carbohydrate.

Nutrition Facts

about 6 servings per container	
Serving size	1 cup (140g)
Amount per serving	
Calories	**170**
	% Daily Value*
Total Fat 8g	10%
Saturated Fat 3g	15%
Trans Fat 0g	
Cholesterol 0mg	0%
Sodium 5mg	0%
Total Carbohydrate 22g	8%
Dietary Fiber 2g	7%
Total Sugars 16g	
Includes 8g Added Sugars	16%
Protein 2g	
Vitamin D 0mcg	0%
Calcium 20mg	2%
Iron 1mg	6%
Potassium 240mg	6%

*The % Dally Value tells you how much a nutrient in a serving of food contributes to a daily diet. 2000 calories a day is used for general nutrition advice.

Example: the label shows that 1 cup of cereal has 22 grams of carbohydrate, but 2 cups of cereal are in the bowl. What are the total grams of carbohydrate?

The answer is 22 grams + 22 grams = 44 grams of carbohydrate.

If the cereal also contains dietary fiber, 2 grams per serving in this example, then the total grams of carbohydrate would be 44 – 4 (2 + 2) = 40 net carbs. This final net carbs total should be used to calculate insulin needs if using insulin-to-carbohydrate ratios (see below).

In the absence of a nutrition label, there are several smartphone applications that can be downloaded to provide nutrition information. Google can be used to find the carbohydrate amount in foods as well as the USDA database.

For most children, a healthy food plan consists of 30–75 grams (2–5 carb choices) at each meal and 10–30 grams (1–2 carb choices) for a snack, more for active teenagers and less for toddlers. Add free foods to meals if desired, but limit to 1–2 servings of free foods (<5 grams of carbohydrate per serving). More than this will have to be added to the total count.

Two Approaches (fixed and flexible): Patients on fixed doses of insulin are prescribed a target of grams of carbohydrates for meals and snacks that they should maintain consistently from day to day. Instead of using carbohydrate exchanges, most patients now use a ratio that represents the amount of carbohydrates (in grams) that 1 U of insulin will cover. This insulin-to-carbohydrate ratio is very individualized, and it is adjusted by trial and error. Nevertheless, the amount of carbohydrate that 1 unit of insulin covers tends to fall after the initial 6-month honeymoon period due to progressive loss of residual endogenous insulin secretion and when patients enter puberty due to increased insulin resistance. The insulin-to-carbohydrate ratio also varies throughout the day, since more insulin is usually needed for breakfast than other meals. Consequently, reasonable accuracy at counting carbohydrates is essential. Unfortunately, we learned from our inpatient studies that many of our teenagers are poor carbohydrate counters.

Low-Carbohydrate Diets

These have had a rebirth in popularity as a result of aggravation with glycemic variability. Most studies of low-carbohydrate diets have been cross-sectional with a lack of control groups, and participants are usually highly motivated individuals who use intensive insulin management practices [9]. An observational study of 1020 Europeans with T1D reported lower HbA1c levels associated with lower carbohydrate intake [5]. However, adherence to restricted diets is challenging over the long term. In adults with T1D, adverse outcomes of very low-carbohydrate/ketogenic diets (<50 grams of CHO or 10% of total calories) include an increased risk of diabetic ketoacidosis, hypoglycemia, dyslipidemia, and glycogen depletion [19]. The safety of low-carbohydrate diets (<130 grams/day or 26% of total energy intake from carbohydrate per ADA definition) has not been established in youth with T1D. Consequently, use of very low-carbohydrate diets in pediatrics should be carefully considered due to potential nutrient deficiencies that may adversely affect growth.

Mixed Meals

Meals made up of carbohydrate and high in dietary fat (like pizza) have been shown to cause late-onset hyperglycemia that lasts for several hours. Wolpert et al. demonstrated that a meal with 50 grams of fat caused significant hyperglycemia over 5 hours despite giving additional insulin [12]. As mentioned before, it has been shown that adding protein to carbohydrate increases glucose. The effect of fat + protein + carbohydrate is cumulative, doubling concentration of glucose at 5 hours [11]. Therefore, pre-meal insulin may need to be calculated based on the content of a meal rather than on the content of carbohydrate alone to reduce post-meal hyperglycemia. Several approaches have been tried such as:

- Giving extra insulin to cover 20 grams of carbohydrate
- Increasing calculated bolus by 20–35%
- Utilizing advance bolus feature in pumps—dual/combo bolus (50%/50%, 60%/40%, or 70%/30%) from 2 to 6 hours

However, no clear effective strategy has emerged as both protein and fat contribute to hyperglycemia and the effect is dose-dependent. Meals very high in fat (i.e., >50 grams) may require double the amount of insulin [12]. Trial and error and continuous glucose monitoring data are the tools to improve meal-related glucose management.

Special Occasions

Children with diabetes can take part in celebrations, just like children without diabetes, but with some adjustments. It is important to determine the timing of the forthcoming event in relation to routine meal time and insulin administration. An extra injection of rapid-acting insulin can be given if the event falls outside of meal time or the injection can be delayed to match the timing of the event. When special foods are the focus of the occasion and the carbohydrate amount exceeds usual intake, additional insulin can be taken, either utilizing an insulin to carbohydrate ratio or giving a few extra units depending on insulin sensitivity. This strategy is preferable, rather than reducing meal carbohydrate intake to accommodate for cake and ice cream. Children with diabetes should not be made feel that they cannot eat the same foods as their peers as this will create feelings of shame and can lead to secretive and disordered eating.

References

1. ISPAD Clinical practice consensus guidelines 2014 compendium. Pediatr Diabetes. 2014;15(Suppl 20):77–85.

2. Smart CE, Annan F, Higgins LA, Jelleryd E, Lopez M, Acerini CL. ISPAD clinical practice consensus guidelines nutritional management in children and adolescents with diabetes. Pediatr Diabetes. 2018;19(Suppl 27):135–53.
3. Aslander-van Vliet E, Smart C, Waldron S. Nutritional management in childhood and adolescent diabetes. Pediatr Diabetes. 2007;8:323–39.
4. Tascini G, Berioli MG, Cerquiglini L, Santi E, Mancini G, Rogari F, Toni G, Esposito S. Carbohydrate counting in children and adolescents with type 1 diabetes. Nutrients. 2018;10:109.
5. Turton JL, Raab R, Rooney KB. Low carbohydrate diets for type 1 diabetes mellitus: a systematic review. Plos One. 2018;e0194987:13.
6. Patton SR, Clements MA, George K, Goggin K. "I don't want them to feel different": a mixed methods study of parents and dietary management strategies for their young child with type 1 diabetes mellitus. J Acad Nutr Diet. 2016;116:272–82.
7. American Diabetes Association medical management of type 1 diabetes. 5th ed. p. 95.
8. Mottalib A, et al. Weight management in patients with type 1 and obesity. Curr Diab Rep. 2017;17:92.
9. Bolla AM, Caretto A, Laurenzi A, Scavini M, Piemonti L. Low carb and ketogenic diets in type 1 and type 2 diabetes. Nutrients. 2019;11:962.
10. Thomas D, Elliott EJ. Low glycaemic index or low glycaemic load, diets for diabetes mellitus. Cochrane Database Syst Rev. 2009;2009(1):CD006296.
11. Smart CEM, Evans M, O'Connell SM, et al. Both dietary protein and fat increase post-prandial glucose excursions in children with type 1 diabetes and the effect is additive. Diabetes Care. 2013;36:3897–902.
12. Wolpert HA, Atakov-Castillo A, Smith SA, Stell GM. Dietary fat acutely increases glucose concentrations and insulin requirements in patients with type 1 diabetes: implications for carbohydrate based bolus dose calculation and intensive diabetes management. Diabetes Care. 2013;36:810–6.
13. Soliman GA. Dietary Fiber, atherosclerosis and cardiovascular disease. Nutrients. 2019;11:1155.
14. Jensen T, Abdelmalek MF, Sullivan S, Nadeau KJ, Green M, et al. J Hepatol. 2018;68:1063–75.
15. Health and Human Services and United States Department of Agriculture. 2020 dietary guidelines for Americans.
16. Silverstein J, Klingensmith G, Copeland K, Plotnick L, Laffel L, et al. Care of children and adolescents with type 1 diabetes: a statement of the American Diabetes Association. Diabetes Care. 2005;28:186–212.
17. Maahs DM, Wadwa RP, Bishop F, Daniels S, Rewers M, Klingensmith G. Dyslipidemia in youth with diabetes: to treat or not to treat. J Pediatr. 2008;153:458–65.
18. Paterson M, Bell KJ, O'Connell SM, Smart CE, Shafat A, King B. The role of dietary protein and fat in glycaemic control in type 1 diabetes: implications for intensive diabetes management. Curr Diab Rep. 2015;15:61.

19. Seckold R, Fisher E, de Bock M, King BR, Smart CE. The ups and downs of low-carbohydrate diets in the management of type 1 diabetes: a review of clinical outcomes. Diabetes Med. 2019;36:326-334.

Suggested Readings

Franz MJ, Boucher JL, Evert AB. Evidenced based nutrition therapy recommendations are effective: the key is individualization. Diabetes Metab Syndr Obes. 2014;7:65–72.

Gökşen D, et al. Effects of carbohydrate counting method on metabolic control in children with type 1 diabetes. J Clin Res Pediatr Endocrinol. 2014;6:74–8.

Reynolds A, Mann J, Cummings J, Winter N, Mete E, Te Morenga L. Carbohydrate quality and human health: a series of systematic reviews and meta-analysis. Lancet. 2019;393:434–45.

Patton S. Adherence to diet in youth with type 1 diabetes. J Am Diet Assoc. 2011;111:550–5.

Laximinarayan S, Reifman J, Edwards S, Wolpert H, Steil GM. Bolus estimation-rethinking the effect of meal fat content. Diabetes Technol Ther. 2015;17:860–6.

Lennerz B, Barton A, Bernstein R, et al. Management of Type 1 diabetes with a very low carbohydrate diet. Pediatrics. 2018;141:e20173349.

Franz MJ, Bantle JP, Beebe CA, Brunzell JD, Chiasson JL, Garg A, Holzmeister LA, Hoogwerf B, Mayer-Davis E, Mooradian AD, et al. Evidenced based nutrition prinicples and recommendations for the treatment and prevention of diabetes and related complications. Diabetes Care. 2002;25:148–98.

Sima P, Vannucci L, Vetvicka V. B-Glucans and cholesterol (review). Int J Mol Med. 2018;41:1799–808.

Erbe JK. Low glycemic index diets for the management of diabetes. Am Fam Physician. 2009;80:941–2.

American Diabetes Association. Children and adolescents: standards of medical care in diabetes. Diabetes Care. 2020;43(Suppl 1):S163–82.

Pańkowska E, Błazik M, Groele L. Does the fat-protein meal increase postprandial glucose level in type 1 diabetes patients on insulin pump: the conclusion of a randomized study. Diabetes Technol Ther. 2012;14:16-22.

Bell KJ, Gray R, Munns D, et al. Estimating insulin demand for protein-containing foods using the food insulin index. Eur J Clin Nutr. 2014;68:1055-1059. https://doi.org/10.1038/ejcn.2014.126.

Bell KJ, Fio CZ, Twigg S, Duke SA, Fulcher G, Alexander K, McGill M, Wong J, Brand-Miller J, Steil GM. Amount and type of dietary fat, post prandial glycemia and insulin requirements in type 1 diabetes: a randomized within subject trial. Diabetes Care. 2020;43:59–66.

Acute Diabetes Complications

10

Ishani Choksi, Shana Mencher, and Anisha Patel

There is much focus on the long-term chronic complications of type 1 diabetes (T1D), especially in youth with T1D due to markedly elevated HbA1c levels in the pediatric age groups (Fig. 10.1). Nevertheless, it is important to recognize that acute complications can be lethal if not identified and managed appropriately. Indeed, diabetic ketoacidosis (DKA), hyperglycemic hyperosmolar state (HHS), and severe hypoglycemia continue to be common, acute threats to the well-being of youth with T1D [1].

Diabetic Ketoacidosis (DKA)

Epidemiology and Risk Factors of DKA

DKA is reportedly the leading cause of morbidity and mortality in pediatric patients with T1D [2]. Many studies have been done to ascertain the incidence of DKA in the pediatric population, as well as identify which factors may place a child at greater risk of devel-

I. Choksi (✉) · S. Mencher · A. Patel
Yale-New Haven Children's Hospital, Department of Pediatrics, Yale School of Medicine, New Haven, CT, USA
e-mail: ishani.choksi@yale.edu; shana.mencher@yale.edu

W. V. Tamborlane (ed.), *Diabetes in Children and Adolescents*, Contemporary Endocrinology,
https://doi.org/10.1007/978-3-030-64133-7_10

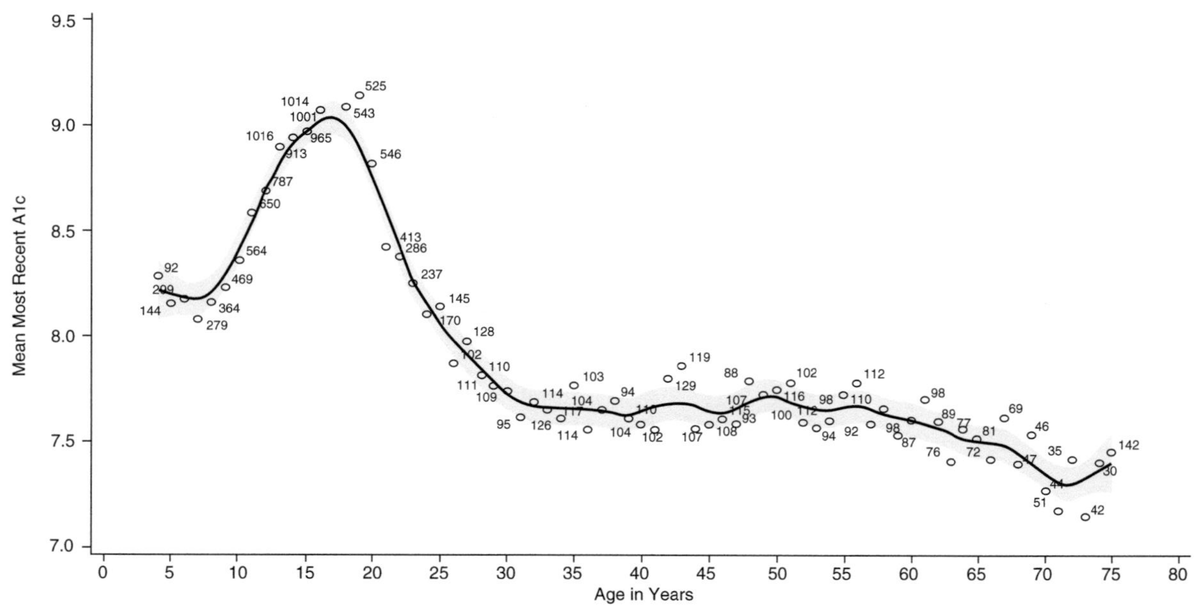

Fig. 10.1 HbA1c levels by age in participants with T1D in the T1D Exchange Registry. (From Miller et al. [1]. Presented with permission)

oping DKA. Based on data from multinational studies of children with newly diagnosed T1D, an estimated 15–70% initially presented in DKA at time of diagnosis [3–5]. Within the United States, between the years 2002 and 2010, SEARCH reported a high, but relatively stable prevalence of DKA at time of diagnosis of T1D in youth aged 0 to 19 years of approximately 30% [4].

Risk factors for presenting in DKA at time of diagnosis include younger age (<5 years), no first-degree relative with T1D, and low socioeconomic status [4]. Among youth with established T1D, DKA remains a common concern. The incidence of DKA in youth with known T1D is reported as between 1 and 10 percent per patient per year [5, 6]. Risk factors for developing DKA in children with established T1D include female gender, ethnic minorities, adolescent age group, HbA1c levels >9.0%, lower household income, no private health insurance coverage, history of previous DKA, difficult family circumstances, and psychiatric disorders [1, 5, 7, 8]. In the United States, patients managing T1D with insulin pumps have a lower DKA rate than those using multiple daily injections (MDIs), but pump site failures are often a cause of DKA [1, 5, 7]. In most cases of DKA in established T1D patients, insulin omission is the cause, whether inadvertently (e.g., pump infusion site failure, limited access to medical care) or intentionally (e.g., psychosocial reasons) [3]. Failure of parents to recognize early signs and symptoms of emerging DKA is another preventable cause of hospitalizations for treatment of severe DKA in children.

Clinical Presentation and Pathophysiology of DKA

Clinical presentation of DKA is variable depending on severity. Symptoms may include nausea and/or vomiting, abdominal pain, dehydration, tachycardia, tachypnea, Kussmaul respiration, blurry vision, and altered mental status [9]. DKA is a catabolic process resulting from underlying insulin deficiency, which can lead to increases in glucagon, catecholamines, cortisol, and growth hormone. Insulin deficiency, as well as increases in counterregulatory hormone levels, leads to increased glucose production by promoting glycogenolysis and gluconeogenesis, decreased glucose utilization, and increased ketone production via lipolysis [3]. Hyperglycemia leads to glucosuria, which ultimately leads to dehydration. Dehydration can cause lactic acidosis and impaired renal function if there is significant volume depletion and poor perfusion [3]. Among the 3 polys (polyuria, polydipsia, and polyphagia), polyphagia is the least likely presenting symptom, because ketosis tends to suppress appetite.

Classification of DKA

The management of DKA depends in large part on the severity of presentation; it can be classified into mild, moderate, or severe. Assuming that T1D patients are not being treated with an SGLT inhibitor, DKA is defined biochemically by the presence of hyperglycemia (blood glucose >200 mg/dL [11 mmol/L]), metabolic acidosis (venous pH <7.3 or serum bicarbonate <15 mmol/L), and ketosis (blood β-hydroxybutyrate ≥3 mmol/L or large ketonuria). Severity of DKA is based on the degree of acidosis [9]:

- Mild: venous pH <7.3 or serum bicarbonate <15 mmol/L
- Moderate: venous pH <7.2, serum bicarbonate <10 mmol/L
- Severe: venous pH <7.1, serum bicarbonate <5 mmol/L

DKA Management

Immediate assessment of vital signs and level of consciousness, and measurement of weight should be performed in all patients with suspected DKA. If clinical signs suggest DKA, biochemical investigation to determine ketone level, blood glucose, electrolytes, and degree of acidemia should promptly ensue. Once diagnosis of DKA is confirmed based on biochemical features and supporting clinical signs, treatment begins with fluid resuscitation based on degree of dehydration. Assessment of dehydration includes evaluating for capillary refill, skin turgor, mucus membranes, pulses, absent tears, and cool extremities [5]. Typically, in moderate DKA, volume deficit is 5–7%, and in severe DKA, approximately 7–10%. In the case of mild DKA with minimal dehydration, therapy can consist of oral fluid hydration and subcutaneous insulin, if the individual is able to tolerate oral fluids [9].

In patients with greater degree of dehydration and DKA severity, IV fluid replacement should begin promptly, even before the initiation of insulin therapy. A normal saline fluid bolus of 10 mL/kg over ~1 hour should be administered first and may be repeated if the patient shows continued signs of poor perfusion/shock. Thereafter, ongoing hydration with IV fluids containing saline (0.45% to 0.9% tonicity), potassium chloride, and either potassium phosphate or potassium acetate should be administered, with a goal of replacing the fluid deficit over 24–48 hours [9]. It is noteworthy that previous studies suggest that neurologic outcomes in children with DKA are not associated with either the rate of IV fluid replacement or the sodium chloride content of the fluids [10].

An intravenous insulin drip should be initiated ~1 hour after starting fluid replacement at a rate of 0.05 to 0.1 units/kg/hour. While not definitively established, an aim is to have blood glucose levels fall gradually at a rate of 50 to 75 mg/dL (2.8–4.2 mmol/L) per hour [5, 9]. However, rapid reductions in blood glucose may be observed due to increasing blood flow to the kidneys with IV hydration. Once blood glucose levels fall below 300 mg/dL (16.7 mmol/L) or if it is falling at a rate faster than 90 mg/dL (5 mmol/L) per hour, dextrose (5%–12.5%) should be added to the IV fluids.

There are often significant derangements of electrolytes in DKA, with changes occurring throughout management. Therefore, electrolytes should be assessed not only at presentation, but also monitored during therapy, as fluid shifts and correction of hyperglycemia will affect serum sodium, potassium, and phosphate levels. Serum sodium levels can be variable with DKA, and often may appear low due to potential dilutional effects of hyperglycemia. Therefore, it is important to calculate a corrected sodium for the degree of hyperglycemia, as shown below [3]:

$$\text{Corrected sodium} = \text{measured Na} + 2 \times \left[\left(\text{plasma glucose mg / dL} - 100 \right) / 100 \right]$$

or

$$\text{Corrected sodium} = \text{measured Na} + 2 \times \left[\left(\text{plasma glucose mmol / L} - 5.6 \right) / 5.6 \right]$$

Even though plasma potassium levels are usually increased with DKA, there is usually depletion of intracellular potassium as a result of extracellular shifts that can be exaggerated by emesis, osmotic diuresis, and a state of secondary hyperaldosteronism causing urinary excretion of potassium [9]. To avoid potential cardiac arrhythmias due to hypokalemia or hyperkalemia, potassium levels should be monitored carefully to ensure adequate replacement. Typically, 20–40 mEq/L is added to IV fluids using a combination of potassium phosphate and either potassium chloride or potassium acetate. Timing of potassium replacement depends on initial potassium concentration: if initially hypokalemic, replacement should be initiated at time of initial rehydration (prior to start of insulin therapy), and if hyperkalemic, potassium should be deferred until serum levels are within normal range and urine output is recorded. If normokalemic at presentation, potassium replacement is still indicated unless there is evidence of renal failure. It is also important to assess an electrocardiogram (ECG) in patients in DKA, especially in circumstances of abnormal potassium measurements. ECG findings in hypokalemia include T-wave flattening and inversion, ST depression, and prolonged PR interval, whereas hyperkalemia results in QT interval shortening and tall, peaked T-waves [9].

Serum phosphate levels are also commonly reduced in DKA due to phosphate losses due to osmotic diuresis and depletion of intracellular phosphate. Phosphate depletion is exacerbated with the initiation of insulin therapy, which promotes phosphate entry into cells [9]. However, adverse effects of severe hypophosphatemia are rare and may be avoided by replacement of phosphate in IV fluids as potassium phosphate [9]. Other electrolyte abnormalities that may occur during DKA treatment include hypocalcemia (especially with phosphate repletion) and hypomagnesemia, and these levels should also be periodically monitored [3].

Metabolic acidosis in DKA is largely due to an anion gap created by ketosis. With adequate fluid and insulin therapy, acidosis is slowly corrected. Insulin works to halt further ketogenesis, promoting keto-acid metabolism and thereby generating bicarbonate [9]. IV fluids help to restore tissue perfusion and renal function, allowing excretion of the organic acids [9]. Several studies have shown that there is no clinical benefit from bicarbonate administration to correct acidosis, and significant adverse effects may result including paradoxical CNS acidosis and hypokalemia from rapid correction of acidosis [3, 5]. Bicarbonate treatment may be indicated only in severe, life-threatening hyperkalemia, severe acidosis (venous $pH < 6.9$), and compromised cardiac contractility [9].

The ultimate goals of therapy in DKA are to correct dehydration and acidosis, suppress ketogenesis, and reduce hyperglycemia [9]. Throughout the management, it is critical that patients are closely monitored, both clinically and biochemically. Patients should have hourly assessments of capillary blood glucoses, vital signs, neurologic status for signs and symptoms of cerebral edema using the Glasgow coma scale, and fluid intake and output. Further laboratory monitoring includes venous blood gases, serum electrolytes, glucose, blood urea nitrogen, serum beta-hydroxybutyrate, creatinine, calcium, magnesium, phosphate, and hematocrit every 2–4 hours, or more frequently if clinically indicated [9]. It is important to note that hyperchloremic metabolic acidosis is often observed during treatment of DKA, resulting from large amounts of chloride in IV fluids and preferential excretion of ketones over chloride in the kidneys [9]. Hyperchloremic metabolic acidosis can be misleading due to an apparent persistence of an increased anion gap; however, measurement of ketones can assist in clarifying the cause of the persistent acidosis. It is usually iatrogenic and resolves spontaneously with appropriate adjustment of IV fluid replacement. Transition to subcutaneous insulin therapy can occur once ketoacidosis has resolved and the patient is able to tolerate oral intake [9].

Close monitoring of patients with DKA is necessary to decrease the morbidity and mortality associated with this condition. Fortunately, the mortality rate in children due to DKA is quite low: reported to be anywhere from 0.15% to 0.30%. Furthermore, the mortality rate may be declining, likely due to increased awareness of symptomatology leading to earlier diagnosis and treatment, increased knowledge of how to manage diabetes and DKA as well as overall improved diabetes treatment and care. Despite low mortality rate, DKA remains the leading cause of death in children diagnosed with T1D under 15 years of age due to delayed recognition of new-onset diabetes by parents, as well as Emergency Department doctors, and failure to recognize early metabolic decompensation in patients with established diabetes. It has also been shown that those with recurrent DKA as well as longstanding poor glycemic control are most at risk for mortality [9]. DKA was also shown to have an adverse impact on brain development in very young children with T1D [11].

Cerebral Edema

Cerebral edema occurs in 0.5 to 0.9% of those in DKA with a mortality rate ranging from 21 to 24%. It is the leading cause of mortality, making up 60 to 90% of all deaths due to DKA. Cerebral injury also accounts for the majority of morbidity due to DKA. Residual deficits can be seen in 10 to 25% of those who survive cerebral edema, which manifests mostly with memory problems [9].

Mental status changes with the Glasgow coma scale (GCS) < 14 can be seen in about 4 to 15% of children who present with DKA. Neuroimaging of children with altered mental status often demonstrates cerebral edema, but it varies in severity and may be subclinical. There are also differing theories to explain the cause of cerebral edema. In the past, it was attributed to fluctuations in serum osmolality due to rapid fluid administration. But, more recently, it is thought that dehydration associated with DKA as well as cerebral hypo-perfusion lead to cerebral injury, which can be exacerbated with treatment. Supporting evidence of this theory stems from the fact that cerebral edema severity does not correlate with initial or change in osmolality, but rather it is associated with the degree of hyperventilation and dehydration. Cases of cerebral edema leading to mortality have shown disruption of the blood-brain barrier, which contributes to the lack of evidence supporting decline in serum osmolality leading to cerebral edema [9].

Risk factors for cerebral edema include those with new-onset T1DM, younger age (<5 years), as well as longer duration of symptoms, which all may be associated with more severe DKA at presentation. Laboratory abnormalities at presentation that pose an increased risk of developing cerebral edema include severe acidosis, increased serum urea nitrogen, and greater degree of hypocapnia after adjusting for degree of acidosis. In terms of treatment; those who receive bicarbonate, are given greater volumes of fluid in the first 4 hours, and are administered insulin in the first hour of treatment with fluids are at higher risk of cerebral edema. In addition, one should be suspicious of cerebral edema in the setting of a significant decrease in serum osmolality early in treatment as well as significant rise in serum sodium or early decline in glucose-corrected sodium during treatment [9].

Cerebral edema is often associated with a headache that begins after initiation of treatment of DKA and may progressively worsen. Cerebral edema may also manifest as altered or change in mental status, including confusion, difficulty arousing, incontinence, or change in behavior. On exam, there may be papilledema or cranial nerve palsies. Cushing's triad is often present later on and is characterized by hypertension, bradycardia, and respiratory depression in the setting of increased intracranial pressure. Cerebral edema can also be associated with hypoxemia. Diabetes insipidus with polyuria and hypernatremia may occur due to cerebral herniation, which disrupts blood flow to the pituitary gland [9].

Treatment of Cerebral Edema

Treatment of cerebral edema should occur promptly once suspected and should include adjusting fluids to maintain normotension and to avoid excessive administration. It is also recommended to decrease intracranial pressure by elevating the head of the bed to 30 degrees. Hyperosmolar agents such as mannitol can be given at a dose of 0.5 to 1 g/kg IV over 10 to 15 minutes, which usually takes effect by 15 minutes and lasts about 2 hours. It can be repeated after 30 minutes if there is no improvement. Hypertonic saline (3%) can be given at a dose of 2.5 to 5 ml/kg over 10 to 15 minutes in addition to mannitol after 15 to 30 minutes or as an alternative to mannitol. In the United States, hypertonic saline has become the more popular choice. If there is any focal neurologic deficit or encephalopathy, neuroimaging should be considered to determine if there is any evidence of hemorrhage or thrombosis that may require intervention. But, again, treatment of cerebral edema should not be delayed so by obtaining imaging [9].

In addition, those who present with new-onset T1D are commonly noted to have impaired cognition acutely, especially in those who present with DKA. A recent study looked at the impact of the severity of DKA on the developing brain in young children ages 4 to 10 years and found that those with moderate or severe DKA had lower scores on IQ testing compared to those without or with mild DKA. In addition, children with moderate or severe episodes of DKA had increased growth pattern in total and regional gray matter volume and white matter volume both at baseline and on repeat neuroimaging (18 months after baseline scan) [11].

Other Complications of DKA

Children with DKA, especially those who have undergone femoral venous catheterization are at risk for deep venous thrombosis, which is thought to be due to the prothrombotic state of DKA. Mild elevations in pancreatic enzymes can be seen in about 40 percent of children in DKA, which is not indicative of acute pancreatitis. If acute pancreatitis is suspected, computed tomography should be performed. Rarer causes of morbidity and mortality include electrolyte derangements, central nervous system complications such as thrombosis or hemorrhage, rhinocerebral or pulmonary mucormycosis, rhabdomyolysis, ischemic bowel necrosis, acute kidney injury, and even renal failure [2].

Hyperglycemic Hyperosmolar State (HHS)

Hyperglycemic hyperosmolar state (HHS) is a condition with severe dehydration accompanied with marked hyperglycemia and hyperosmolarity usually without ketoacidosis. However, HHS can be accompanied by DKA, namely, HHS or combined DKA-HHS. In adults with hyperglycemic crisis, approximately one third of each condition was seen with respective increases in mortality [12]. Presentation of HHS in children and adolescents has increased since the 1960s with associated increases in obesity and type 2 diabetes [13]. In pediatrics, presentation of HHS usually accompanies new-onset diabetes; however, adults can present with a known history of diabetes. Mortality in pediatrics has been reported to be between 10% and 37% [13, 14].

HHS is most commonly seen in adults with poorly controlled type 2 diabetes and limited epidemiological data is available in pediatrics. Existing evidence has shown that African American adolescents and those with new-onset diabetes more frequently present with HHS [12, 14]. In addition, individuals with T1D and infants with neonatal diabetes can also develop HHS. Individuals who presented with HHS frequently had family history of T2D and acanthosis nigricans. In addition, approximately 20% had a preexisting history of limited cognitive function or mental illness [12]. Therefore, risk factors for HHS include obesity, T2D, and children treated with atypical antipsychotics [15].

Due to a lack of symptoms of abdominal pain, vomiting, hyperventilation, polyuria and polydipsia, HHS may be asymptomatic, and the associated metabolic derangement may go unrecognized until severe dehydration [9]. Children may present with a more severe degree of dehydration without identifiable precipitating factors. Moreover, individuals with components of DKA and HHS have been reported to have a higher mortality rate than DKA or HHS alone [12]. Indeed, the only newly diagnosed patient with diabetes who died during initial treatment at Yale was determined to have DKA-HHS rather than DKA alone. The ultimate cause of death in that teenager was delayed correction of severe fluid and electrolyte depletion due marked hyperglycemia.

Pathophysiology of HHS

Insulin deficiency/resistance along with glucagon excess leads to development of DKA and HHS and other exacerbating factors include catecholamine, growth hormone and cortisol secretion, which contribute to increase in blood glucose and ketones [16]. In DKA, insulin deficiency is more severe; whereas, mild insulin presence helps decrease lipolysis and ketogenesis but not hyperglycemia in HHS. The more severe hyperglycemia in HHS contributes to higher plasma osmolality, which rapidly increases due to the large volume of urinary electrolyte loses driven by hyperglycemia. Severe dehydration in HHS is also accompanied by electrolyte abnormalities including hypokalemia, hypophosphatemia, hypomagnesemia, and hypocalcemia can also contribute to increased morbidity and mortality in HHS [16].

Criteria for HHS alone includes the following: plasma glucose concentration >600 mg/dL (33.3 mmol/L); venous pH > 7.25; arterial pH > 7.30; serum bicarbonate>15 mmol/L; small ketonuria, absent to mild ketonemia; effective serum osmolality>320 mOsm/kg; and altered consciousness (e.g., obtundation, combativeness) or seizures [9].

HHS Management

Management in children and adolescents has been adopted from the adult experience. The recommendation is to focus on correcting dehydration and normalization of sodium to decrease osmolality. Initially isotonic saline bolus of >20 mL/kg should be given, with correction of fluid deficit over the first 24–48 hours. As with DKA, if there is rapid decline in blood glucose concentrations (i.e., >90 mg/dL or >5 mmol/L per hour) addition of 2.5–5% dextrose containing fluid should be considered. In the setting of poor circulatory volume, urinary losses should be replaced with sodium-containing fluids. Patients with HHS also have severe potassium deficiency, which could be exacerbated by early and rapid treatment with insulin. Rapid shift in potassium is correlated with cardiac arrhythmias, and therefore potassium replacement should start once plasma potassium levels are normal. Volume repletion, decline in hyperglycemia, and osmolality usually occur with fluid resuscitation alone, and initiation of insulin treatment is delayed until glucose no longer decreases with fluid alone; usual stating dose of 0.025–0.05 units/kg/hr of regular insulin. If more severe ketoacidosis is present, insulin should be started earlier; however, insulin bolus is not recommended. (ISPAD guidelines) [9].

Complications of HHS

While organ failure due to delayed rehydration is an ever present danger with HHS [13], other mineral deficiencies are also common, including phosphate and magnesium. However, bicarbonate treatment is contraindicated. Phosphate and magnesium can both directly affect calcium levels and therefore should be adequately corrected with replacement. Another complication associated with HHS is an increased risk of venous thrombosis, especially with central vein catheterizations. In pediatric patients, heparin treatment should be reserved for those requiring central venous catheters or are immobilized for greater than 24–48 hours. Rhabdomyolysis is another complication, which can be associated with acute kidney failure along with mineral abnormalities and exaggerated increases in blood glucose. Altered mental status is common, but it is not usually associated with cerebral edema. Although malignant hyperthermia has rarely been reported in pediatric patients with HHS, it is associated with high mortality [9].

Hypoglycemia

Severe hypoglycemia and DKA are the two most common acute complications of T1D [1]. Hypoglycemia is largely an iatrogenic complication that remains an important limiting factor in maintaining optimal glycemic control in an individual. An important example was the sharp increase in the frequency of severe hypoglycemic events in well-controlled participants in the DCCT study [17]. More recently, several studies have shown that advances in diabetes technologies have increased the frequency of achieving near normal blood glucose levels in a greater percentage of youth with T1D without increasing the frequency of hypoglycemia. However, technological advancements such as sensor-augmented insulin pump therapies and continuous glucose monitors (CGMs) have not eliminated the risk of severe hypoglycemic events. Indeed, hypoglycemia in T1D continues to be a potentially fatal complication that necessitates an understanding of its underlying pathophysiology to provide further insight into identifying risk factors and in developing prevention strategies.

Definition and Classification of Hypoglycemia in Diabetes

One definition of clinically important hypoglycemia is those events that result in reductions in plasma glucose and cognitive impairments that require the assistance of another person for treatment [18]. A biochemical definition is a reduction in plasma glucose to values <54 mg/dL. However, patients with poorly controlled T1D may have a higher glycemic threshold at which they experience hypoglycemic symptoms, whereas patients with well-controlled T1D and/or recent or recurrent hypoglycemic events may experience hypoglycemic symptoms at a lower plasma glucose concentration [19]. With the increased availability of continuous glucose monitoring, consensus conferences have established the target range of optimal glucose values as between 70 and 180 mg/dL (3.9–10.0 mmol/L), and the diagnosis of hypoglycemia at <54 mg/dL or <3.0 mmol/L.

Epidemiology/Frequency of Hypoglycemia

It is difficult to determine an exact incidence of hypoglycemia, as mild hypoglycemia events, especially those that are asymptomatic, are very common in the T1D population and often are unrecognized and underreported [20]. Moreover, prior to the development of CGMs, very limited data were available regarding hypo- and hyperglycemia during the overnight period. It has only recently been established that nighttime is the worst time because glucose control is so variable from one night to the next. While Albert Einstein defined insanity as doing the same thing over and over again and always expecting a different result, we define insanity in T1D as taking the same overnight basal insulin dose over and over again and always getting a different result. Recent prospective and retrospective observational studies have assessed the incidence of severe hypoglycemia in pediatric patients with T1D. These studies indicate that there has been a significant reduction in the incidence of severe hypoglycemia events and that low HbA1c is no longer associated with severe hypoglycemia [21]. Nevertheless, the T1D Exchange Clinic Registry data indicate that severe hypoglycemia events continue to be a problem with youth with T1D [1]. They found that severe hypoglycemia was more common in the younger age group, with 9.6% of participants experiencing severe hypoglycemia in the 2–6-year-old age group versus 6.9% in the 18–26-year-old age group [8].

Risk Factors of Hypoglycemia

The risk factors for hypoglycemia in T1D ultimately stem from a relative and/or absolute insulin excess and are intensified due to a compromised physiologic response to falling blood glucose levels [5]. Absolute insulin excess occurs when insulin doses are ill-timed, the incorrect type, or there is decreased clearance of insulin as in the case of renal failure [5]. Relative insulin excess is the result of decreased exogenous glucose influx (fasting periods such as overnight, less food consumption), increased glucose utilization (exercise), decreased endogenous glucose production (alcohol ingestion), and increased insulin sensitivity [20]. It is important to consider potential comorbidities when hypoglycemia is recurrent, such as hypothyroidism, celiac disease, and Addison's disease, as well as potential psychological distress [20].

Hypoglycemia-Associated Autonomic Failure (HAAF)

Recurrent hypoglycemia events in an individual with T1D are often associated with impaired awareness of hypoglycemia, also known as hypoglycemia-associated autonomic failure (HAAF). Other risk factors for HAAF include recent antecedent hypoglycemia, prior exercise, and sleep [22]. In non-diabetic individuals, the temporal physiologic responses to falling plasma glucose concentrations are as follows: (1) a decrease in insulin, (2) an increase in glucagon, and (3) an increase in epinephrine [5]. In T1DM, endogenous insulin secretion is absent for the most part, and glucagon responses to insulin-induced hypoglycemia are typically lost early in the course of diabetes [20]. Thus, sympatho-adrenal responses remain the only defense against hypoglycemia in youth with T1D, but recurrent hypoglycemia episodes lead to delayed and/or attenuated sympatho-adrenal responses and a 25-fold increased risk of severe hypoglycemia [5]. It has also been shown that children with and without T1D have impaired sympatho-adrenal responses to hypoglycemia during sleep at night [23].

Treatment of Hypoglycemia

Hypoglycemia is generally quickly ameliorated by consuming 15 grams of rapidly absorbed carbohydrates, typically in the form of glucose tablets or fruit juice with resolution seen in approximately 15 minutes. This is known as the "rule of 15" and if hypoglycemia persists after 15 minutes, consumption of another 15 grams of carbohydrate should be repeated. It is important to follow up treatment with a snack or meal after blood sugar has risen to a level of >70 mg/dL (>3.9 mmol/L), since treatment with carbohydrate alone leads to a short-lived rise in glucose that wears off by 2 hours [20]. Severe hypoglycemia accompanied by cognitive impairment requiring assistance by another person can be treated with glucose gel or icing administered to the buccal mucosa or even sublingually, which is rapidly absorbed in the case of a child refusing oral treatment.

The recently approved intra-nasal glucagon powder [23] and pre-mixed glucagon for injection are highly effective. These two new glucagon preparations can replace previous injectable preparations that were unstable in solution and required multiple steps prior to injection. Patients with severe hypoglycemia in a hospital setting can receive intravenous glucose, either 10% or 20% for a total of 200 to 500 mg/kg of glucose in total. It is also important to educate caregivers that after a severe episode of hypoglycemia, their child is at risk of another event, especially in the subsequent 24 hours. Therefore, alterations in insulin therapy and decrease in total daily dose of insulin by at least 10–20% is appropriate [20].

Complications of Hypoglycemia

In pediatrics, acute complications of hypoglycemia include altered level of consciousness, seizures, and even mortality (e.g., "dead in bed syndrome"). Transient decline in cognitive function can be seen both with hyperglycemia and hypoglycemia in young children with diabetes, but long-term cognitive dysfunction in the setting of hypoglycemia is thought to be unlikely. In fact, the Diabetes Research in Children Network (DirecNet) has reported that chronic hyperglycemia may lead to a greater impairment of brain growth and development in very young children than hypoglycemia [11]. One of the most common fears of caretakers and children alike is nocturnal hypoglycemia.

While none of the patients in our program has been found to be dead in bed due to nocturnal hypoglycemia, fear of hypoglycemia can have a significant impact on psychological morbidity of children and caregivers, leading to poorer glycemic control as they accept higher glucose levels, especially overnight. Indeed, parents of very young children with T1D seem to use CGM devices exclusively as a means to prevent hypoglycemia rather than to improve overall glycemic control. Other adverse effects of fear of hypoglycemia include decreased quality of life and increased parental burden in managing their child's diabetes [20]. Having very young children with T1D use a continuous glucose monitoring device with “share” capabilities has become increasingly popular with parents, because they can follow their child’s sensor glucose levels remotely.

Prevention of Hypoglycemia

Even with the most meticulous diabetes control, it is nearly impossible to prevent hypoglycemia, although frequency and severity can be significantly minimized with use of newer technology, adequate education to predict such events (e.g., vigorous exercise in the afternoon resulting in nocturnal hypoglycemia on the following night), and the ready availability of methods to treat hypoglycemia. Education should focus on recognizing other risk factors such as decreased oral intake, change in insulin regimen, and alcohol intake in young adults. It is important for those with T1D to always be prepared with a rapid-acting glucose source as well as to wear a medical alert to identify others if they were to be found unconscious from a severe hypoglycemic episode. Education in teenage years should focus on effects of alcohol on blood sugar levels as well as importance of blood glucose testing prior to driving to avoid motor vehicle accidents due to hypoglycemia. It is important to note that it may be difficult for very young children to verbalize symptoms of hypoglycemia, and therefore the caretaker must recognize any change in behavior may be due to a low blood sugar level [20]. A very promising feature in prevention and reduction of hypoglycemia has been the recent FDA approval of the first hybrid closed-loop systems that can automatically adjust between meal and overnight infusion rates of insulin pumps based on real-time variations in sensor glucose levels. As noted above, standalone CGM equipped with remote monitoring capabilities are very popular with parents of very young children [20].

The ultimate goal in diabetes management is to obtain the best glycemic control, while simultaneously reducing the risk of hypoglycemia. Therefore, one must individualize HbA1c and glycemic goals based on risk factors and history of severe hypoglycemia. More recently, attention has been focused on increasing time in range and minimizing hypoglycemia, especially severe hypoglycemia to ensure hypoglycemia awareness. This can be achieved through proper education as well as increased utilization of newer technology.

References

1. Miller KM, Foster NC, Beck RW, Bergenstal RM, DuBose SN, DiMeglio LA, Maahs DM, Tamborlane WV, T1D Exchange Clinic Network. Current state of type 1 diabetes treatment in the U.S.: updated data from the T1D Exchange clinic registry. Diabetes Care. 2015;38:971–8.
2. Glaser N. Treatment and complications of diabetic ketoacidosis in children and adolescents. Uptodate. 2019, January 18. Accessed 17 March 2020.
3. Wolfsdorf J, Glaser N, Sperling MA. American Diabetes Association. Diabetic ketoacidosis in infants, children, and adolescents: a consensus statement from the American Diabetes Association. Diabetes Care. 2006;29:1150–9.
4. Dabelea D, Rewers A, Stafford JM, Standiford DA, Lawrence JM, Saydah S, Imperatore G, D'Agostino RB Jr, Mayer-Dvavis EJ, Pihoker C. SEARCH for Diabetes in Youth Study Group. Trends in the prevalence of ketoacidosis at diabetes diagnosis: the SEARCH for Diabetes in Youth Study. Pediatrics. 2014;133:e938–45.
5. Schlomo M, Koenig R, Rosent C, Aucus R, Goldfine A. Williams textbook of endocrinology. 14th ed. Philadelphia: Elsevier, Inc.; 2020.
6. Rewers A, Chase HP, Mackenzie T, Walravens P, Roback M, Rewers M, Hamman RF, Klingensmith G. Predictors of acute complications in children with type 1 diabetes. JAMA. 2002;287(19):2511–8.
7. Maahs DM, Hermann JM, Holman N, et al. Rates of diabetic ketoacidosis: international comparison with 49,859 pediatric patients with type 1 diabetes from England, Wales, the U.S., Austria, and Germany. Diabetes Care. 2015;38(10):1876–82.
8. Cengiz E, Xing D, Wong JC, et al. Severe hypoglycemia and diabetic ketoacidosis among youth with type 1 diabetes in the T1D exchange clinic registry. Pediatr Diabetes. 2013;14(6):447–54.
9. Wolfsdorf JI, Glaser N, Agus M, Fritsch M, Hanas R, Rewers A, Sperling MA, Codner E. ISPAD clinical practice consensus guidelines 2018: diabetic ketoacidosis and the hyperglycemic hyperosmolar state. Pediatr Diabetes. 2018;19:155–77.
10. Kuppermann N, Ghetti S, Schunk JE, Stoner MJ, Rewers A, McManemy JK, Myers SR, Nigrovic LE, Garro A, Brown KM, Quayle KS, Trainor JL, for the PECARN DKA FLUID Study Group. Clinical trial of fluid infusion rates for pediatric diabaetic ketoacidosis. NEJM. 2018;378(24):2275–87.

11. Aye T, Mazaika PK, Mauras N, Marzelli MJ, Shen H, Hershey T, Cato A, Weinzimer S, White NH, Tsalikian E, Jo B, Reiss AL. for the Diabetes Research in Children Network (DirecNet) Study Group. Impact of early diabetic ketoacidosis on the developing brain. Diabetes Care. 2018;
12. Pasquel FJ, Tsegka K, Wang H, Cardona S, Galindo RJ, Fayman M, Davis G, Vellanki P, Migdal A, Gujral U, Narayan VKM, Umpierrez GE. Clinical outcomes in patients with isolated or combined diabetic ketoacidosis and hyperosmolar hyperglycemic state: a retrospective, hospital-based cohort study. Diabetes Care. 2020;43(2):349–57.
13. Rosenbloom AL. Hyperglycemic hyperosmolar state: an emerging pediatric problem. J Pediatr. 2010;156(2):180.
14. Canarie MF, Bogue CW, Banasiak KJ, et al. Decompensated hyperglycemic hyperosmolarity without significant ketoacidosis in the adolescent and young adult population. J Pediatr Endocrinol Metab. 2007;20:1115–1124– 20, 1115–1124.
15. Kharode I, Coppedge E, Antal Z. Care of children and adolescents with diabetes mellitus and hyperglycemia in the inpatient setting. Curr Diab Rep. 2019;19:85.
16. Hirsch IB, Emmett M. Diabetic ketoacidosis and hyperosmolar hyperglycemic state in adults: Epidemiology and pathogenesis. Up to date Mar 2020, Topic 1794 Version 15.0.
17. Hypoglycemia in the diabetes control and complications trial. The diabetes control and complications trial research group. Diabetes. 1997;46(2):271–86.
18. Defining and reporting hypoglycemia in diabetes. American Diabetes Association workgroup on hypoglycemia. Diabetes Care. 2005;28(5):1245–9.
19. Seaquist ER, Anderson J, Childs B, et al. Hypoglycemia and diabetes: a report of a workgroup of the American Diabetes Association and the Endocrine Society. J Clin Endocrinol Metab. 2013;98(5):1845–59.
20. Abraham MB, Jones TW, Naranjo D, Karges B, Oduwole A, Tauschmann M, Maahs DM. ISPAD clinical practice consensus guidelines 2018: assessment and management of hypoglycemia in children and adolescents with diabetes. Pediatr Diabetes. 2018;27:178–92.
21. Cherubini V, Rabbone I, Lombardo F, et al. Incidence of severe hypoglycemia and possible associated factors in pediatric patients with type 1 diabetes in real-life, post-Diabetes Control and Complications Trial setting: a systematic review. Pediatr Diabetes. 2019;20(6):678–92.
22. Jones TW, Porter P, David EA, O'Leary P, Stick S, Fraser F, Sherwin RS, Tamborlane WV. Suppressed epinephrine responses during sleep: a contributing factor to the risk of nocturnal hypoglycemia in insulin-dependent diabetes. N Engl J Med. 1998;338:1657–62.
23. Sherr JL, Ruedy KJ, Forster N, et al. Glucagon nasal powder: a promising alternative to intramuscular glucagon in youth with type 1 diabetes. Diabetes Care. 2016;39:555–62.

Sick Day Management

11

Shana Mencher, Ishani Choksi, and Anisha Patel

The Challenge

The Type 1 Diabetes (T1D) Exchange Registry has shown that diabetic ketoacidosis (DKA) remains a serious threat to youth with T1D, especially those with chronic poor diabetes control [1]. It is imperative that parents of children with T1D who develop acute symptoms of nausea, abdominal pain or discomfort, and (especially) vomiting remember that these are the cardinal signs of evolving diabetic ketoacidosis (DKA). They must also know that they need to closely monitor their child for elevated blood sugar levels, as well as blood β-hydroxybutyrate or urine ketone levels that signal the development of DKA. Most of all, they need to realize that DKA can develop with *or* without the presence of another acute illness such as a viral or bacterial infection. Unfortunately, parents often forget the threat of DKA until acidosis and dehydration result in a hospital admission to the pediatric intensive care unit: outcomes that could be avoided in most patients.

S. Mencher (✉) · I. Choksi · A. Patel
Yale-New Haven Children's Hospital, Department of Pediatrics, Yale School of Medicine, New Haven, CT, USA
e-mail: shana.mencher@yale.edu; shani.choksi@yale.edu; anisha.patel@yale.edu

W. V. Tamborlane (ed.), *Diabetes in Children and Adolescents*, Contemporary Endocrinology,
https://doi.org/10.1007/978-3-030-64133-7_11

Sick Day Management

In terms of recurrent DKA, the only way to prevent another episode is to identify the underlying cause, which is most commonly due to insulin omission, whether purposeful or not. At a minimum, education should be given to all families regarding prevention of DKA on an annual basis. DKA events occur all too often because families have forgotten the early warning signs of deterioration of metabolic control of diabetes. One of our mothers was once asked why she did not call sooner when her child with T1D vomited for the 6th time in 5 hours. She said, "his sister was sick with the flu and I thought he had the same thing." Another parent said, "I've never had to check ketones before; we haven't had any test strips for years, anyway." DKA prevention should be reinforced more frequently in high-risk groups (e.g., adolescents) with longer duration of T1D, with poor glycemic control and in disadvantaged minority families [2].

More often than not, there is a psychosocial cause of insulin omission, and multidisciplinary efforts should include a social worker as well as provide mental health resources if necessary. One should also consider an eating disorder and omitting insulin to try to lose weight, especially in adolescents and young adults with T1D. In addition, parental abuse or neglect in the form of inadequate parental supervision, mental health disease such as depression, or inability to pay for diabetes supplies should be considered and ameliorated if possible. It has been shown that parental administration of insulin can reduce frequency of recurrent DKA by as much as tenfold [3]. Modest improvements in overall glycemic control have also been shown by administration of long-acting basal insulin during the school week by school personnel.

Patients who are managed with an insulin pump most commonly present in DKA due to lack of recognition of hyperglycemia as a sign of an infusion site failure, resulting in the failure to replace the site and/or give insulin via an injection. Paradoxically, the T1D Exchange Registry has reported that the frequency of DKA is lower in youth being treated with an insulin pump than by insulin injection therapies. However, this difference may simply represent greater awareness of the dangers of DKA by parents of youth on insulin pumps [2].

As a reminder, urine ketone strips only measure urinary concentrations of acetoacetate, and even modest elevations in β-hydroxybutyrate levels can be associated with high urinary acetoacetate levels. Moreover, β-hydroxybutyrate is not measured in the urine, even though markedly elevated β-hydroxybutyrate levels cause most of the complications of DKA. It has also been shown that measurements of blood β-hydroxybutyrate levels instead of urinary ketone levels decrease both emergency department visits and hospitalizations by providing more precise determinations of the degree of metabolic deterioration than measuring urine ketones [4].

DKA is often triggered by an infection, which makes early metabolic deterioration even harder to recognize, especially in youth with chronically poor glycemic control. In most cases, this represents a situation in which patients already have unmet insulin needs that are exaggerated by an intercurrent infection. It is also not surprising that some youngsters with T1D feel safer in the hospital than at home, and "forgetting" to take their insulin provides a means to be hospitalized. When directly questioned why a youngster with T1D ended up in the PICU, the most common answer is "I forgot to take my insulin"; be it either by injection or by pump. The best way to really know how often an adolescent has missed a dose of insulin is to ask the number of doses she/he has missed during the past week. It is surprising that such a straightforward question often results in a straight answer. Unfortunately, even with proper education and access to a provider 24 hours a day for emergencies, preventable DKA events in youth with T1D occur all too often.

In addition to reducing morbidity and mortality, developing programs to prevent DKA would have a major economic impact in reducing healthcare costs due to hospitalizations. It is estimated that the United States alone spends ~$90 million annually to treat DKA. If we could reduce the number of cases of DKA by 10%, this could save nearly $10 million annually [2]. While the morbidity and mortality rates with DKA are small, almost every adverse outcome of DKA in pediatrics is followed by an expensive and protracted lawsuit, which adds greatly to the adverse economic impact of these DKA events.

Studies that have examined the prevention of DKA at diagnosis of T1D have mostly focused on improving community education and awareness. There was a highly successful poster campaign in schools in Parma, Italy, which also provided local pediatricians with means to measure glycosuria and blood glucose leading to a significant reduction in DKA in comparison to other local communities. Some limitations included a small sample size and high rate of DKA prior to intervention. In Australia, a similar education campaign with posters proved successful. On the other hand, similar studies showed no benefit in Wales and Austria. Therefore, limited evidence exists that widespread community education can reduce DKA incidence in new-onset T1D. It is recommended that efforts to do so should focus on simple messages that are clear and relevant [5].

Sick Day Guidelines

The basic principles of sick day management and DKA prevention are frequent monitoring of blood glucose and ketones (i.e., β-hydroxybutyrate) and access to the diabetes team 24 hours a day, 7 days a week. Specifically, blood glucose (and ketones) should be monitored at least every 2–4 hours, but continuous glucose monitoring of sensor glucose levels may provide a clearer view of early metabolic decompensation. When faced with early signs of DKA, parents should be encouraged to call the diabetes team for advice in diabetes management. As a preemptive approach to guide our parents with T1D children, we have provided them with a take-home visual flowchart (see Fig. 11.1 below), which has resulted in improved recognition of DKA symptoms as well as better sick day management. This brief educational intervention has resulted in fewer emergency department visits and alternatively more frequent use of emergency diabetes telephone line for assistance [6].

Ketosis is due to increased lipolysis and ketogenesis, which is a sign of absolute or relative insulinopenia and elevated

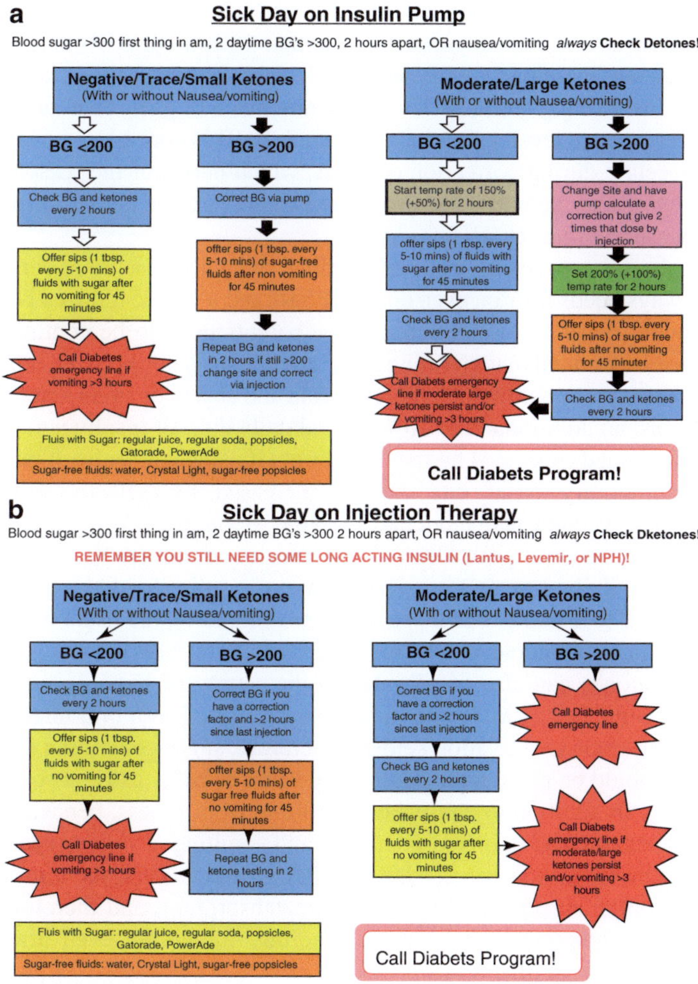

Fig. 11.1 Sick day management using (**a**) insulin pump (**b**) injection therapy

counterregulatory hormones commonly seen in illness due to stress and/or fever. There are three different types of ketones: acetoacetate (which is measured by urine test strips), acetone (which often produces a distinctive, fruity odor to the patient's breath), and β-hydroxybutyrate (BHB) (which is measured by blood ketone strips). It is important to note that the ratio of BHB to acetoacetate increases significantly during the development of ketoacidosis (e.g., blood BHB levels are much higher than urine acetoacetate levels). On the other hand, BHB is converted to acetoacetate during correction of DKA, which is one of the reasons why urinary ketones take so long to clear (i.e., urine ketone strips measure *only* acetoacetate) [4].

It is important to educate families annually that their child always needs insulin, even during illness and it can be reduced but should never be stopped. Similarly, parents need to be continuously reminded that vomiting is a sign of ketosis until proven otherwise. In the setting of hyperglycemia and absent or small ketone levels, an additional 5 to 10% of total daily dose of insulin is recommended every 2–4 hours. In addition, if using an insulin pump, a temporary basal rate can be increased by ~10 to 30%. Hyperglycemia and moderate or large ketones are serious and highly concerning for DKA. Therefore, an additional 10 to 20% of total daily dose as a correction dose of insulin should be given every 2 to 4 hours. For those on an insulin pump, the usual basal insulin infusion rate can be increased by ~20 to 50% [4].

Ketones can also be elevated in the setting of hypoglycemia when one has a gastroenteritis or other cause of poor oral intake, which leads to starvation ketosis. Therefore, sugar-containing fluids should be given with insulin, which has to be adjusted accordingly. In addition to nausea and vomiting from illness, persistent ketosis can lead to increased nausea and vomiting: a vicious cycle that increases the risk for DKA. After gastroenteritis, there may be continued poor oral intake and malabsorption, and therefore blood sugar levels need to be carefully monitored even after recovery from illness [4].

The other essential component of management is fluids. Families should have a variety of fluids on hand including those containing sugar and those that are sugar-free, as well as fluids with adequate electrolytes. If blood sugars are >200 mg/dL, it is recommended to give small sips of sugar-free beverages if no emesis in past 30–45 minutes, but if blood sugars are <200, then sugar-containing beverages should be given [4, 6]. If a patient develops ketosis and hyperglycemia on an insulin pump, one should assume there is an infusion site failure, and the infusion site needs to be changed. In addition, to ensure the child receives insulin, it is recommended to administer a correction dose via an injection. Basal insulin infusion rates may need to be adjusted by 20 to 50% in either direction depending on blood glucose and ketone levels [4].

Recognizing DKA When Treated with Sodium-Glucose Transport Protein 2 (SGLT) Inhibitors

It is important to understand that ketogenesis can be common in certain situations such as in patients who consume low carbohydrate diets, those afflicted by disordered eating behaviors, and those on SGLT2 or SGLT1/2 inhibitors. Although SGLT inhibitors have not yet been approved by the US FDA as adjunctive treatments of children, adolescents, and adults with T1D, they have been used "off-label" in adults with T1D. In a recent study [7], we examined the early metabolic changes in a small number of adults with T1D following shutting off their insulin pumps before and after treatment with a SGLT2 inhibitor (Canagliflozin). Our data demonstrated that treatment with a SGLT2 inhibitor did not increase the rate of ketogenesis following the interruption of the basal insulin infusion. Rather, the failure of patients to recognize early metabolic decompensation relates to a much more gradual rise in plasma glucose levels (Fig. 11.2). Moreover, turning ketogenesis off during rescue treatment with insulin was not adversely affected by SGLT2 inhibitor treatment [8]. Therefore, frequent monitoring of glucose and blood β-hydroxybutyrate levels is always recommended in patients receiving treatment with this class of drug.

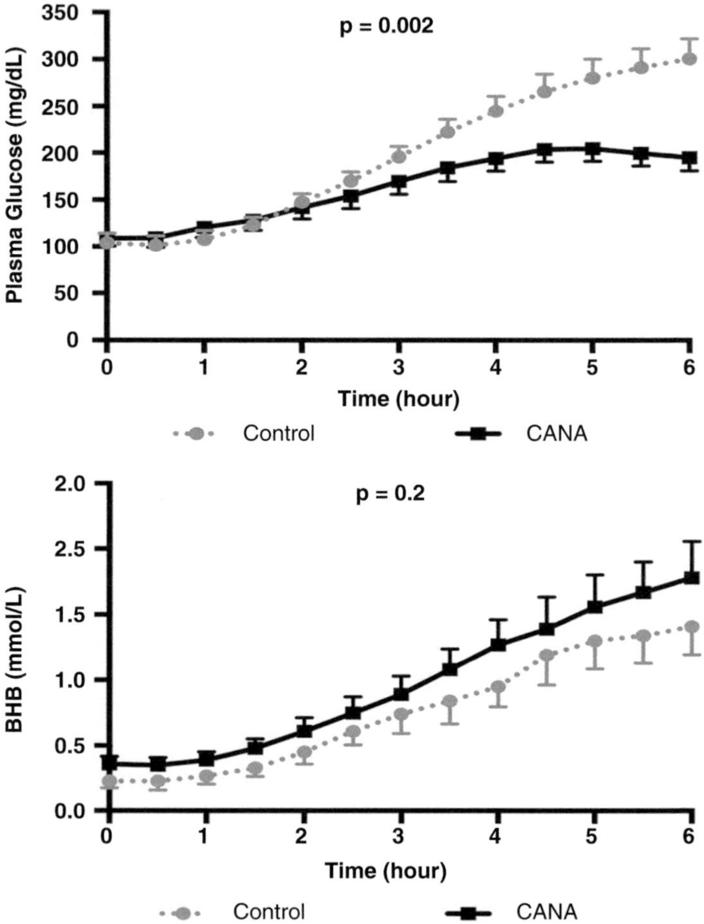

Fig. 11.2 Delayed increases in plasma glucose but not β-hydroxybutyrate during treatment with a SGLT2 inhibitor (Canagliflozin) versus a pretreatment control study. (From Patel et al. [7]. Reprinted with permission from the publisher, Mary Ann Liebert, Inc.)

References

1. Cengiz E, Xing D, Wong J, Beck RW, Haymond MW, Miller KM, Rewers A, Seiple DL, Shanmugham S, Tamborlane WV, Willi SM. Wolfsdorf JI for the T1D Exchange Clinic Network. Risk of severe hypoglycemia and diabetic ketoacidosis and associated risk factors among youth with type 1 diabetes in the T1D exchange registry cohort. Pediatr Diabetes. 2013;14:447–54.
2. Maahs DM, Hermann JM, Holman N, Foster N, Kapellen T, Allgrove J, Schatz DA, Hofer SE, Campbell F, Steigleder-Schweiger C, Beck RW, Warner JT, Holl RW. On behalf of the National Paediatric Diabetes Audit & the Royal College of Paediatrics & Child Health (UK), the DPV initiative (Germany and Austria), and the T1D Exchange Clinic Network (US). Rates of diabetic ketoacidosis: international comparison with 49,859 pediatric patients from England, Wales, the United States of America, Austria and Germany. Diabetes Care. 2015;38:1876–82.
3. Wolfsdorf JI, Glaser N, Agus M, Fritsch M, Hanas R, Rewers A, Sperling MA, Codner E. ISPAD clinical practice consensus guidelines 2018: diabetic ketoacidosis and the hyperglycemic hyperosmolar state. Pediatr Diabetes. 2018;19:155–77.
4. Laffel LM, Limbert C, Phelan H, Virmani A, Wood J, Hofer SE. ISPAD clinical practice consensus guidelines 2018: sick day management in children and adolescents with diabetes. Pediatr Diabetes. 2018;19:193–204.
5. Jeffries CA, Nakhla M, Derraik JGB, Gunn AJ, Daneman D, Cutfield WS. Preventing diabetic ketoacidosis. Pediatr Clin N Am. 2015;62:857–71.
6. Vitale RJ, Card C, Lichtman JH, Weyman K, Michaud C, Sikes K, Tamborlane WV, Weinzimer SA. Effectiveness of a diabetic ketoacidosis prevention intervention in children with type 1 diabetes. SAGE Open Nurs. 2018;4:1–6.
7. Patel N, Van Name M, Carria L, Cengiz E, Weinzimer S, Tamborlane WV, Sherr J. Altered patterns of early metabolic decompensation in type 1 diabetes during treatment with a SGLT-2 inhibitor: an insulin pump suspension study. Diabetes Technol Ther. 2017;19:618–22.
8. Siebel S, Galderisi A, Patel NS, Carria LR, Tamborlane WV, Sherr JL. Reversal of ketosis in type 1 diabetes is not adversely affected by SGLT2 inhibitor therapy. Diabetes Technol Ther. 2019;21:101–4.

Screening for Comorbidities and Complications of T1D

12

Michelle Van Name, Patricia Gatcomb, Elizabeth A. Doyle, and William V. Tamborlane

Background In the pre-DCCT era, youth with type 1 diabetes (T1D) suffered from a variety of early vascular complications. While intensive insulin therapy has markedly delayed or prevented the development of these early complications, young patients whose control is suboptimal on their current treatment are still susceptible to micro- and macrovascular complications. Moreover, the presence of one endocrine disorder (i.e., T1D) increases the risks of other endocrine disorders and screening for these comorbidities are recommended in youth with T1D.

M. Van Name (✉) · P. Gatcomb · W. V. Tamborlane
Yale-New Haven Children's Hospital, Department of Pediatrics, Yale School of Medicine, New Haven, CT, USA
e-mail: michelle.vanname@yale.edu; patricia.gatcomb@yale.edu

E. A. Doyle
Yale School of Nursing, Primary Care Division, Orange, CT, USA

W. V. Tamborlane (ed.), *Diabetes in Children and Adolescents*, Contemporary Endocrinology,
https://doi.org/10.1007/978-3-030-64133-7_12

Associated Autoimmune Diseases

- Autoimmune thyroid disease is the most common disorder associated with T1D. We measure TSH levels at the time of diagnosis of T1D, since a substantial percentage of patients have thyroid dysfunction either before or at the time of diagnosis of diabetes [1]. However, thyroid function tests may be misleading at the time of diagnosis. Consequently, obtaining TSH and thyroid hormone levels tend to be more accurate if follow-up studies are obtained during the honeymoon period, once satisfactory glycemic control is achieved. If testing is normal, follow-up studies should be performed every 1–2 years. A simple TSH test can be obtained annually during a routine, follow-up diabetes clinic visit, with more extensive testing if TSH levels are elevated or suppressed.
- Celiac disease is also a common comorbidity of T1D but, like thyroid disease, screening for celiac disease at the time of diagnosis can give artifactually abnormal results. However, initial screening for celiac disease should be undertaken relatively early during T1D [2]. Standard screening tests include measurement of tissue transglutaminase IgA if serum IgA is in range or deaminated gliadin antibodies and tissue transglutaminase IgG. Biopsy or additional testing in collaboration with pediatric gastroenterology can confirm the diagnosis. Children with confirmed celiac disease should be placed on a gluten-free diet. Periodic rescreening of patients in whom initial screening negative is recommended but the optimal frequency of rescreening is unclear.
- The trio of T1D, autoimmune thyroid disease, and adrenal insufficiency, (autoimmune polyglandular syndrome type 2, formerly called Schmidt's syndrome) has been reported, but the development of adrenal insufficiency in T1D is relatively uncommon. However, we have a few patients with this syndrome. In some cases, hyperpigmentation due to markedly elevated ACTH levels led to their diagnoses.

Macrovascular Complications of T1D Although cardiovascular disease is very uncommon in adolescents and young adults with

T1D, blood pressure should be measured at every face-to-face clinic visit, and a fasting lipid profile should be obtained after diagnosis when glycemia has improved. If LDL is <100 mg/dl, testing should be repeated at 9–11 years of age. If lipids are abnormal, medical nutrition therapy in addition to optimizing glycemic control are the first steps in treatment. If LDL is <100 mg/dL, repeat screen every 3 years is sufficient [3]. Urine albumin/creatinine ratio (ideally morning sample) should be obtained annually in patients with a duration of diabetes >5 years and who have started puberty or reached 10 years old. Treatment (e.g., an ACE inhibitor) should be considered if 2 of 3 repeat samples over 6 months' time indicate elevated albumen/creatinine ratios [3]. It is noteworthy, however, that in many participants in the DCCT/EDIC study, elevated albumin/creatinine ratios normalized without requiring treatment.

Retinopathy Since poor glycemic control of T1D can lead to asymptomatic microvascular disease that may warrant treatment, regular screening for diabetic retinopathy in youth with T1DM has been recommended in the past. Currently, the American Diabetes Association advises annual retinopathy screening to begin once a child is 11 years of age or has started puberty, and has been diagnosed with T1D for 3–5 years. Eye exams every 2 years or even less frequently have also been suggested as acceptable depending on the clinical scenario [3].

Annual evaluation may have been appropriate in the pre-intensive treatment era, when markedly elevated HbA_{1c} levels were associated with the very early development and rapid progression of diabetic retinopathy. However, results of the Diabetes Control and Complications Trial (DCCT) demonstrated that improved glycemic control with intensive treatment in adolescents markedly delays early microvascular changes in the retina. Since HbA_{1c} levels in youth with T1DM are lower now than they were 30–40 years ago, the yield from such screening examinations are also likely to be reduced, raising the question of whether screening guidelines for retinopathy should be adjusted further.

To evaluate this question in adolescents with T1D, we retrospectively reviewed the results of eye examinations carried out as part of the Diabetes Control and Complications Trial in all participants who were between 13 and 17 years of age at randomization into that study [4]. Every 6 months, participants had standardized 7-field fundus photographs between 1983 and 1993, and transitions in retinopathy status were evaluated over this time period. The 195 participants had a median baseline HbA1c level of 9.3% and had an average of 5.3 retinopathy assessments during the average 2.3 years of study follow-up while under 18 years of age. None of the participants developed severe non-proliferative diabetic retinopathy or proliferative retinopathy. This clinical trial evidence suggests that in youth <18 years of age with T1D, frequent eye exams may not be universally necessary. Indeed, for most of youth with an initial screen of no diabetic retinopathy or even mild non-proliferative retinopathy, a single screening eye exam may be enough before 18 years of age (Table 12.1). Moreover, only one pediatric participant in DCCT developed clinically significant macula edema (CSME) (image b, Fig. 12.1) during the initial 6 moths of the study. However, there was a substantial resolution of CSME after 12 months in the study without any treatment.

Psychological Screening Screening for disordered eating, depression, anxiety, and diabetes distress are also recommended for adolescents and young adults with T1D [3]. However, no consensus exists on which measures are optimal, and most previous

Table 12.1 Observed number of transitions of the retinopathy status from one visit to the next visit among the 195 adolescent participants while still less than 18 years of age

From → to	No DR	Mild NPDR	Moderate NPDR	Severe NPDR	PDR	CSME
No DR	393	105	1	0	0	0
Mild NPDR	83	230	9	0	0	1
Moderate NPDR	0	9	3	0	0	0
Severe NPDR	0	0	0	0	0	0

There were 1031 retinopathy assessment visits in the 195 participants from 13 to <18 years of age

Abbreviations: *CSME* clinically significant macular edema, *DR* diabetic retinopathy, *NPDR* non-proliferative diabetic retinopathy

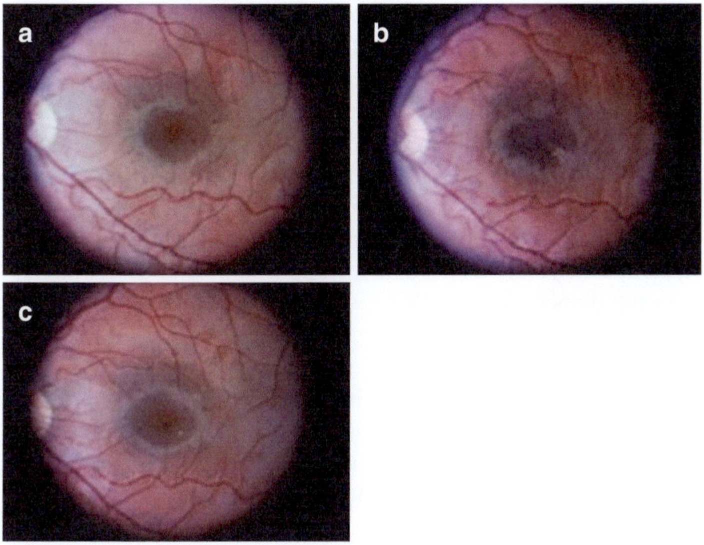

Fig. 12.1 Spontaneous correction of clinically significant macular edema without treatment (image **c**) in the only teenager who had potentially treatable retinopathy on second eye exam (image **b**) indicates a normal macula (image **a**)

studies have used non-specific measures. In our clinical program, screenings for these disorders in adolescents and young adults have used two disease-specific measure and one general measure at the time of transition from pediatric to adult care.

Disordered Eating We were particularly interested in determining the prevalence and clinical characteristics of disordered eating behaviors (DEBs) in young adult males and females with T1D screened during transition from pediatric to adult diabetes care. DEBs were measured with the diabetes-specific Diabetes Eating Problem Survey–Revised (DEPS-R). In this study, 27 females and 33 males (aged 21 ± 2.5 years) completed the DEPS-R. Of these, 27% of females and 18% of males gave evidence of disordered eating behaviors, and DEPS-R scores correlated with increased BMI values. These findings support the contention that clinicians should assess for DEB in both male and female adolescents and young adults with T1D, especially overweight patients with poor glycemic control [5].

Depressive Symptoms and Diabetes Distress In a descriptive study of young adults with T1D in our practice, 16.7% of our sample had depressive symptoms and 20.9% had diabetes distress. Of those noted to have symptomatic depression or diabetes distress as adolescents, several subsequently screened negative on transition to adult care. It is also noteworthy that depression and diabetes distress positively correlated with glycated hemoglobin (HbA1c) levels. These data indicate that formal screening of adolescents and young adults provide opportunities to detect depression and diabetes distress [6].

Anxiety Symptoms of anxiety, as well as anxiety-related disorders are common in patients with diabetes [7]. Providers should consider screening for anxiety in patients who exhibit excessive concerns regarding complications, fear of hypoglycemia, and taking their insulin or other medications [8].

References

1. Roldan MB, Alonso M, et al. Thyroid autoimmunity in children and adolescents with type 1 diabetes. Diabetes Nutr Metab. 1999;12:27–31.
2. Holmes GKT. Screening for coeliac disease in type 1 diabetes. Arch Dis Child. 2002;87:495–8.
3. American Diabetes Association. 13. Children and adolescents: standards of medical care in diabetes-2020. Diabetes Care. 2020;43(Suppl 1):S163–82.
4. Gubitosi-Klug RA, Bebu I, White NH, Malone J, Miller R, Lorenzi GM, Hainsworth DP, Trapani VR, Lachin JM, Tamborlane WV, Diabetes Control and Complications Trial (DCCT)/Epidemiology of Diabetes Interventions and Complications (EDIC) Research Group. Screening eye exams in youth with type 1 diabetes under 18 years of age: Once may be enough? Pediatr Diabetes. 2019;20:743–9.
5. Doyle EA, Quinn S, Ambrosino J, Weyman K, Tamborlane WV, Jastreboff A. Disordered eating behaviors in emerging adults with type 1 diabetes: not just a female problem. J Pediatr Health Care. 2017;31:327–33.
6. Quinn SM, Ambrosino JM, Doyle EA, Weyman K, Tamborlane WV, Jastreboff AM. Utility of screening for psychological problems during transition of care in young adults with type 1 diabetes. Endocr Pract. 2016;22:1104–10.

7. Smith KJ, Beland M, Clyde M, et al. Association of diabetes with anxiety: a systematic review and meta-analysis. J Psychosom Res. 2013;74(2):89–99.
8. American Diabetes Association. Standards of medical care in diabetes. Diabetes Care. 2016;39(Suppl 1):S86–93.

Adjunctive Therapies for Type 1 Diabetes

13

Laura Nally, Michelle Van Name, William V. Tamborlane, and Jennifer Sherr

Background

It can be argued that little has changed in the treatment of T1D since insulin was introduced in the 1920s. Yes, we have many new insulin preparations, much better ways to monitor the effectiveness of insulin with current blood glucose meters and new continuous glucose monitors and improved ways to deliver insulin with insulin pumps and semi-automatic hybrid closed-loop insulin delivery systems. However, the basic pharmacology has not changed: it has always been all about insulin, insulin, and more insulin. That is why many clinicians who care for patients with T1D are excited about the possibilities of using the plethora of new anti-diabetic drugs that have been approved for use in adults withT2D, as adjunctive agents to insulin in the treatment of

L. Nally (✉) · M. Van Name · W. V. Tamborlane · J. Sherr
Yale-New Haven Children's Hospital, Department of Pediatrics, Yale School of Medicine, New Haven, CT, USA
e-mail: laura.nally@yale.edu

W. V. Tamborlane (ed.), *Diabetes in Children and Adolescents*, Contemporary Endocrinology,
https://doi.org/10.1007/978-3-030-64133-7_13

T1D. Unfortunately, pramlintide is rarely used in T1D, metformin has not been found to be of benefit youth with T1D, and other new T2D drugs have not been approved for use in adults and children with T1D by the FDA. Despite these limitations, we discuss each of the potential adjunctive treatments below. In addition, Table 13.1 summarizes the benefits, potential uses, cautions, and side effects of adjunctive therapies for type 1 diabetes [1].

Table 13.1 Benefits, potential uses, cautions, and side effects of adjunctive therapies for type 1 diabetes

Adjunctive therapy	Benefits	Potential use	Cautions	Side effects
Pramlintide (Amylin analog)	↓ A1c, weight loss	↓ Post-prandial hyperglycemia	Worsening of gastroparesis, caution in those with hypo unawareness	Nausea, vomiting, anorexia, headache
Metformin	Modest ↓ A1c and weight	Obese/ overweight patients with T1D	Lactic acidosis, B12 deficiency, may require decreases in insulin doses to avoid hypos	Diarrhea, nausea/ vomiting, abdominal discomfort, headache
Liraglutide (GLP1-agonist)	Weight reduction, lower insulin doses	Obese/ overweight patients with T1D	Risk of thyroid cancer, pancreatitis	Nausea, diarrhea, vomiting, ↓appetite, dyspepsia, constipation
SGLT2 and SGLT1/2 inhibitors	↓ A1c, weight loss, lower TDD insulin	Patients with T1D knowledgeable on signs/ symptoms of ketosis, willing to check ketone levels regularly, and are aware of risk of DKA	Euglycemic DKA, ↓ insulin doses to avoid hypoglycemia	Polyuria, risk of DKA

From Nally et al. [1]

Pramlintide

Pramlintide is an analog of amylin which is co-secreted with insulin by β-cells in response to blood sugar elevations. When amylin is secreted, it slows gastric emptying, inhibits glucagon release from α-cells in the pancreatic islets, and promotes centrally mediated satiety. Pramlintide is the only adjunctive therapy that has been FDA approved for use in T1D based on the results of pivotal, randomized phase III studies, which showed that pramlintide lowered A1c by ~0.5%. Furthermore, its use is associated with weight loss in overweight or obese patients; a mechanism that is similar to amylin. As shown in Fig. 13.1, treatment with pramlintide slows gastric emptying and reduces peak post-prandial plasma glucose levels. The putative effect of pramlintide is that it suppresses meal-stimulated increases in plasma glucagon, which, in turn, mitigates post-prandial hyperglycemia. We have shown that these actions of pramlintide persist over time; whereas, similar actions by liraglutide wane very quickly (Fig. 13.1).

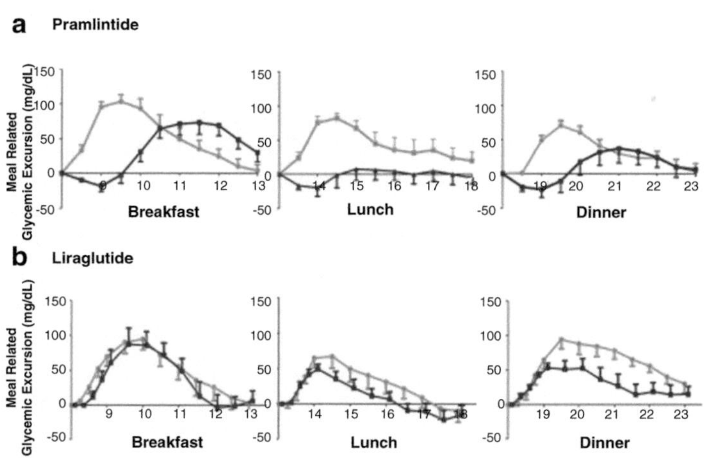

Fig. 13.1 Delayed absorption and reductions in post-prandial peaks of glucose following treatment with pramlintide compared to liraglutide. (From Sherr et al. [2])

Even though it was approved by the FDA in 2005, very few patients with T1D are currently being treated with pramlintide. The major obstacle to widespread use of this agent is that it requires additional 3–4 subcutaneous injections per day, which has proven too cumbersome for many patients. While co-formulation of pramlintide and insulin have been considered, no combination product has yet to be developed and commercialized.

Metformin

Metformin was approved for adults with T2D in 1994 and in children with T2D in 1999. In clinical practice, it is occasionally used "off-label" as an adjunctive therapy for T1D, especially in patients who are overweight or obese. However, evidence suggests that it has marginal benefits at best in lowering A1c levels in T1D. For example, in a systematic review of metformin as an adjunctive treatment in adults with T1D, it was associated with a statistically significant reduction in total daily insulin dose (i.e., ~6.6 units/day), but not lowering of A1c. However, there was insufficient data at that time to determine the efficacy of metformin in obese pediatric patients with T1D.

To fill the gap in the efficacy of metformin use in adolescents with T1D, Yale was part of a multi-center study of the efficacy of metformin as adjunctive treatment of overweight/obese adolescents with T1D [3]. This study represented the largest pediatric trial in youth with T1D, and it was carried out by centers in the Type 1 Diabetes Exchange (T1DX). In that study, 140 overweight adolescents with T1D were randomized to adjunctive treatment with metformin or placebo. While there were modest reductions in body weight and total daily doses of insulin in the metformin group after 26 weeks, there was no difference in A1c levels (Table 13.2). On the other hand, hypoglycemia and gastrointestinal side effects were more common with metformin. This study indicates that there is little benefit of metformin as adjunctive therapy to improve glycemic control in T1D.

Table 13.2 Lack of substantial benefit of metformin on lowering of HbA1c in obese adolescents with T1D

	Metformin	Placebo	*P* value*
Baseline	*N* = 71	*N* = 69	
HbA1c – *Mean ± SD*	8.8% ± 0.8%	8.8% ± 0.7%	
13 weeks	*N* = 68	*N* = 68	
HbA1c – *Mean ± SD*	8.7% ± 1.0%	8.9% ± 1.0%	
Change from baseline to 13 weeks – *Mean ± SD*	−0.2% ± 0.8%	0.1% ± 0.8%	
Mean adjusted difference (95% CI)	−0.30% (−0.56%, −0.03%)		0.02
HbA1c decrease ≥0.5% – *% (95% CI)*	29% (18%, 41%)	29% (18%, 41%)	0.95
HbA1c increase ≥0.5% – *% (95% CI)*	18% (8%, 27%)	28% (17%, 39%)	0.18
26-weeks	*N* = 70	*N* = 69	
HbA1c – *Mean ± SD*	9.0% ± 1.0%	8.9% ± 1.1%	
Change from baseline to 26 weeks – *Mean ± SD*	0.2% ± 0.8%	0.2% ± 0.9%	
Mean adjusted difference (95% CI)	0.01% (−0.26%, 0.29%)		0.93
HbA1c decrease ≥0.5% – *% (95% CI)*	19% (8%, 28%)	26% (15%, 37%)	0.27
HbA1c increase ≥0.5% – *% (95% CI)*	44% (32%, 56%)	35% (23%, 46%)	0.21

*Only *P* values ≤0.05 indicate statistically significant differences between the metformin and placebo groups

Glucagon-Like Peptide 1 (GLP1) Receptor Agonists and Dipeptidyl Peptidase-4 (DPP-4) Inhibitors

GLP-1 is a peptide hormone secreted from the endocrine L-cells in the intestine in response to ingesting a meal. Like amylin, GLP-1 slows gastric emptying, inhibits glucagon release, and reduces appetite. GLP-1 is rapidly degraded by DPP-4, making its half-life extremely short. GLP-1 receptor agonists, including liraglutide, were developed to maintain a longer half-life in the circulation than native GLP-1, namely, ~13 hours.

In a randomized, double-blind placebo controlled trial in 40 normal weight participants with suboptimal control of T1D, patients in the liraglutide treatment group had an overall reduction in A1c that was not significantly different than what was seen in the placebo group. In other studies of GLP-1 agonist treatment, participants with T1D have reported some lowering of insulin doses and body weight, but no significant changes in the frequency of hypoglycemic events or lowering of A1c levels. As noted above, we have shown that the ability of GLP-1 agonists to slow gastric emptying and inhibit glucagon secretion wanes rapidly during treatment of T1D (Fig. 13.1). This may explain why improved metabolic control of T1D was not observed. Since loss of appetite and weight loss may be the only benefits of GLP-1 agonists as adjunctive treatments for T1D, studies to gain regulatory approval for this indication are not being pursued by industry. It is noteworthy that treatment with GLP1-agonists during the honeymoon phase of T1D, during which many retain clinically significant residual endogenous insulin secretion, has not been studied.

Since GLP-1 agonists appear to provide little benefit besides appetite suppression and weight loss in insulin-deficient patients with T1D, it is predictable that DPP-4 inhibitors would have even less benefit, since they are weight neutral when used in treating T2D. Thus, it is not surprising that two meta-analysis of randomized controlled trials DPP-4 inhibitors showed no effect on A1c levels.

Sodium-Glucose Cotransporter-2 Inhibitors (SGLT2*i*) and Sodium-Glucose Cotransporter-1/2 Inhibitors (SGLT-1/2*i*)

The kidneys play a key role in regulating glucose levels in the body. In the proximal tubule, sodium glucose cotransporters mediate the transfer of 90% of glucose from the lumen back into the bloodstream. Consequently, by inhibiting SGLT-2 and preventing the reabsorption of glucose in the nephron, increased glucose is lost as glucosuria and plasma glucose levels are reduced.

Using this insulin-independent mechanism, there is the potential to reduce hyperglycemic exposure, while simultaneously reducing body weight. In view of these benefits, several drugs in this class have been approved for use in adults with T2D. It is also noteworthy that studies in adults with T2D have shown that SGLT2*i* had beneficial effects on heart failure and cardiovascular mortality.

Several groups have evaluated the efficacy and safety of SGLT2*i* in adults with T1D. In two meta-analyses of trials with SGLT2*i* as adjunctive therapy for adults with T1D involving 21 clinical trials and >5,000 patients, these agents lowered A1c, body weight, daily doses of insulin, and blood pressure. CGM studies showed decreased average glucose levels and lower glucose variability.

Nevertheless, enthusiasm for use of SGLT2i has been dampened by reports of "euglycemic DKA" in patients with both T1D and T2D. Since T1D patients using insulin pumps are at substantial risk for DKA because they do not take long-acting insulin and they often experience infusion site failures, we have recently shown that early metabolic decompensation resulting in increased circulating β-hydroxybutyrate levels during treatment of T1D with SGLT2*i* is not due to accelerated ketogenesis. What was observed was a slow and blunted rise in plasma glucose levels, undoubtedly due to increased urinary glucose excretion.

In current clinical practice, few T1D patients routinely measure blood β-hydroxybutyrate or urine ketone levels; instead, they rely on marked and persistent elevations in plasma glucose to recognize impending DKA. A recent consensus conference on mitigating the risks of DKA in patients treated with SGLT2*i* emphasized the need to monitor blood β-hydroxybutyrate levels regularly and to recognize the early symptoms of elevated ketone levels, namely, nausea, abdominal discomfort, and vomiting. Unfortunately, too many T1D patients fail to recognize that blood β-hydroxybutyrate levels are increasing even in the absence of SGLT2*i* treatment. Thus, the benefits of SGLT2*i* treatment in T1D may not be worth the risks, at least in the subset of poorly controlled patients who may need these drugs the most. On the other hand, it is possible by teaching patients on these therapies to be diligent with blood β-hydroxybutyrate and urine ketone testing; these agents can successfully be employed in the treatment of both T1D and T2D.

Combined SLGT-1/2 inhibitors are currently undergoing FDA evaluation for the treatment of T1D. SGLT-1/2*i* not only prevents reabsorption of glucose in the kidneys but also inhibits glucose absorption from the small intestine. Interestingly, SGLT1-mediated glucose transport in the kidney is activated when the glucose exceeds the ability of the SGLT2 to reabsorb glucose. The studies to date suggest that with careful patient selection and education regarding a slightly higher risk of DKA, SGLT-1/2i's can provide metabolic health benefits to those with T1D. Unfortunately, the US FDA has not approved any SGLT2*i* or SGLT1/2*i* for use in adults with T1D. Without an indication for use of these agents in adults with T1D, pharmaceutical companies have put a hold on pivotal randomized clinical trials of these agents in youth with T1D.

References

1. Nally LM, Sherr JL, Van Name M, Patel A, Tamborlane WV. Pharmacologic treatment options for type 1 diabetes: What's new? Expert Rev Clin Pharmacol. 2019;12:471–9.
2. Sherr JL, Patel NS, Michaud CI, Palau-Collazo MM, Van Name MA, Tamborlane WV, Cengiz E, Carria L, Tichy E, Weinzimer SA. Mitigating meal-related glycemic excursions in an insulin sparing manner during closed loop insulin delivery: the beneficial effects of adjunctive pramlintide and liraglutide. Diabetes Care. 2016;39:1127–34.
3. Libman LM, Miller KM, DiMeglio LA, Bethin KE, Katz M, Shah A, Simmons J, Haller MJ, Raman S, Tamborlane WV, Coffey J, Saenz A, Beck RA, Nadeau KJ for the T1D Exchange Clinic Network Metformin RCT Study Group. A randomized trial of metformin as an adjunct therapy for overweight adolescents with type 1 diabetes. JAMA. 2015;314:2241–50.

Exercise and Diabetes 14

Jasmine Gujral, Melinda Zgorski,
and William V. Tamborlane

Exercise and Diabetes

Regular exercise and active participation in organized activities have positive implications for both the psychosocial and physical well-being of all children and are especially important for children with diabetes. Exercise and being physically fit are associated with increased sensitivity to insulin and enhanced glucose utilization. Moreover, lowering plasma glucose by encouraging exercise provides an important alternative to simply increasing insulin doses in youth with T1D who are not optimally controlled.

Despite its many benefits, exercise in children with diabetes can make it more challenging to regulate glucose levels. The Diabetes Research in Children Network (DirecNet) study, in which Yale participated, demonstrated that antecedent exercise in the afternoon increased the risk of nocturnal hypoglycemia on the following night by twofold [1] (Fig. 14.1). In a subsequent

J. Gujral (✉) · M. Zgorski · W. V. Tamborlane
Yale-New Haven Children's Hospital, Department of Pediatrics,
Yale School of Medicine, New Haven, CT, USA
e-mail: jasmine.gujral@yale.edu

W. V. Tamborlane (ed.), *Diabetes in Children and Adolescents*, Contemporary Endocrinology,
https://doi.org/10.1007/978-3-030-64133-7_14

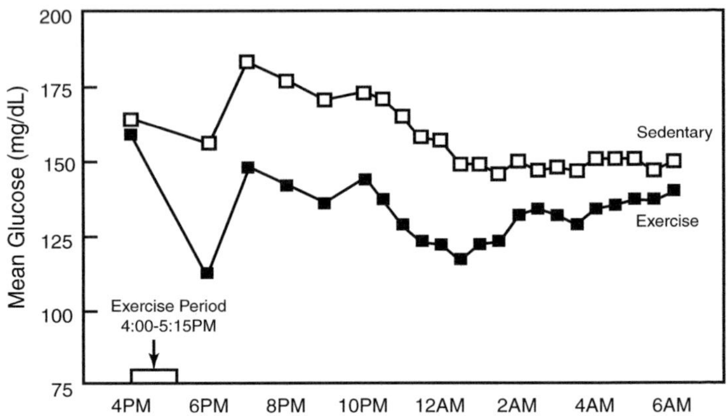

Fig. 14.1 Mean glucose levels in youth with T1D on the exercise and sedentary days. (From: The DirecNet Study Group [1], with permission)

Australian study, McMahon and colleagues showed that the delayed fall in plasma glucose following afternoon exercise typically occurs up to 7–11 hours later [2], namely, during sleep at night. This effect is compounded by the intermittent and spontaneous nature of physical activity in children, especially those not involved in organized sports or activities.

As many children participate in late afternoon or evening activities, a reduction in the dose of overnight insulin may help to prevent the delayed hypoglycemia during the subsequent night. As in many other diabetes-related activities, the magnitude of the reduction of overnight insulin following afternoon exercise is often a matter of trial and error that differs from one individual to the next and from one night to the next. This is one of the reasons why nighttime is the worst time for diabetes. It is also why hybrid closed-loop insulin delivery systems that can automatically adjust the rate of overnight insulin delivery based on changes in sensor glucose values are so attractive to so many. With these devices, nighttime no longer needs to be the worst time for parents of children with T1D.

Children with T1D who participate in any type of exercise should test their blood glucose values before, during, and after the exercise. When working with children and their families, it is important to discuss the triad of exercise, food intake, and insulin. When exercise is increased, one of the others must be adjusted to minimize the risk of hypoglycemia. For patients on injections of insulin, the dose of insulin can be reduced when exercise is planned; otherwise, additional snacks may need to be eaten. In patients who use insulin pump therapy, suspension of the basal infusion rate (or simply disconnecting the pump) during exercise can reduce the risk of hypoglycemia [3]. Use of temporary basal rates during and after exercise can help to prevent hypoglycemia during the activity and later that day or night. Serious athletes may need to reload on carbohydrates following intense and/or prolonged activity in addition to adjusting their insulin doses. Some patients find that raw cornstarch can slow the digestion of sugar, providing a more sustained fast-acting carbohydrate effect in combatting exercise-induced nocturnal hypoglycemia.

We recently undertook an assessment of the efficacy of whether snacking could be used with a closed-loop (CL) insulin delivery system to avoid exercise-induced reductions in plasma glucose, as well as elevations in plasma glucose at the end of exercise. To address this issue, 12 adolescent and young adult participants with T1D (age 13–36 years, diabetes duration 10.7 ± 8.4 years, and A1c 7.4% ± 0.8%) underwent two 105-min exercise studies, one with and one without snacking. Exercise, which commenced at 3 PM, consisted of four 15-min periods of brisk treadmill walking separated by three 5-min rest periods, followed by a 30-min recovery period. Fifteen to 30 grams of carbohydrate (Gatorade) was provided on snacking visits just before and midway through the exercise period. Plasma glucose and insulin were measured every 15–20 min during the exercise studies.

Baseline glucose levels were similar for CL alone (164 ± 16 mg/dL) versus CL+ snack (172 ± 11 mg/dL). However, during exercise, plasma glucose levels fell by 53 ± 10 mg/dL without snacking versus a modest 10 ± 13 mg/dL increase in plasma glucose with snacking; similar differences in the change in circulating glucose levels were observed at the end of recovery period. Hypoglycemia requiring rescue treatment during exercise occurred in three non-snacking visits versus none with snacking

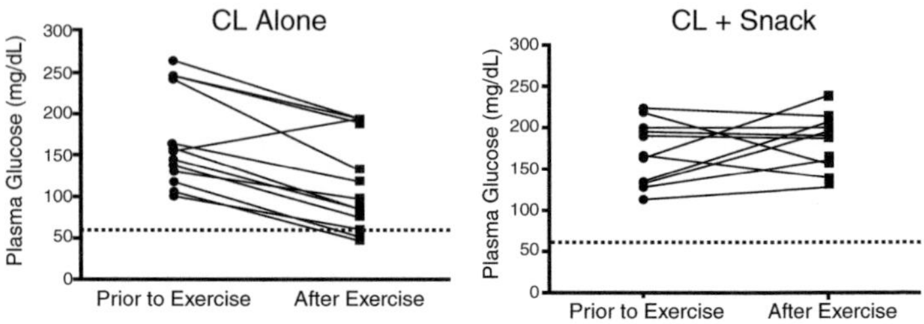

Fig. 14.2 Plasma glucose levels before and at the end of exercise sessions in individual subjects. Each participant is represented by a single line indicating change in glucose level from the start to the end of the exercise period. The dashed line represents the threshold to define hypoglycemia (60 mg/dL). (From: Patel et al. [4], with permission)

(Fig. 14.2). These results support the use of a simple snacking strategy to avoid exercise-induced lowering of plasma glucose while on CL insulin delivery. Since full CL insulin delivery is not yet approved for use in T1D, trial and error are still key components in the management of exercise and glucose levels in children with diabetes.

References

1. The Diabetes Research in Children Network (DirecNet) Study Group. Impact of exercise on overnight glycemic control in children with type 1 diabetes. J Pediatr. 2005;147:528–34.
2. McMahon SK, Ferreira LD, Ratnam N, et al. Glucose requirements to maintain euglycemia after moderate-intensity afternoon exercise in adolescents with type 1 diabetes are increased in a biphasic manner. J Clin Endocrinol Metab. 2007;92:154–68.
3. The Diabetes Research in Children Network (DirecNet) Study Group. Prevention of hypoglycemia during exercise in children with type 1 diabetes by suspending basal insulin. Diabetes Care. 2006;29:2200–4.
4. Patel NS, Van Name MA, Cengiz E, Carria LR, Tichy EM, Weyman K, Weinzimer SA, Tamborlane WV, Sherr JL. Mitigating reductions in glucose during exercise on closed loop insulin delivery: the Ex-Snacks Study. Diabetes Technol Ther. 2016;18:794–9.

15

Psychosocial Challenges of Diabetes

Elizabeth A. Doyle, Amy Page, and Kathryn Nagel

Introduction

Diabetes is an insidious condition; it requires patients and their families to be "on" 24 h per day, 7 days per week. Consequently, it can have a profound negative impact on lifestyle and interpersonal relationships between parents and their children with diabetes, since all burdens of diabetes and its care are superimposed on the already challenging transitions through childhood, adolescence, and into early adulthood. Moreover, other children in the family may suffer from feelings of neglect, due to the greater attention paid to their sibling with diabetes.

These issues are not unique to T1D but are observed in families with children with other chronic disorders of childhood and adolescence. Such stresses are often exaggerated in families in which the parents are separated or divorced, as well as those with low

E. A. Doyle (✉)
Yale School of Nursing, Primary Care Division, Orange, CT, USA
e-mail: elizabeth.doyle@yale.edu

A. Page
Yale Children's Hospital, Social Work, New Haven, CT, USA

K. Nagel
Yale New Haven Hospital, Internal Medicine/Pediatrics Residency, New Haven, CT, USA

W. V. Tamborlane (ed.), *Diabetes in Children and Adolescents*, Contemporary Endocrinology,
https://doi.org/10.1007/978-3-030-64133-7_15

income and language and cultural barriers. Indeed, one of our teenage patients complained to her parents that she was tired of being in an intact family, since her friends could play one divorced parent against the other. Difficulties between parents and patients often result in nonadherence to making good food choices, missing premeal boluses of insulin, skipping blood glucose meter testing, and not using continuous glucose monitoring devices. Similarly, deliberate omissions of insulin doses to limit weight gain are often pleas for psychological help. Feelings of being different or alone are also common. In addition, a surprising number of parents are delighted to turn over exclusive responsibility for management of diabetes to their children with T1D.

The most common responses that we receive from teenagers who miss a lot of premeal insulin doses are "I forget" or "I guess I'm lazy" or "I'm always late for school." The truth is that most teenagers who have long-standing diabetes are just tired of having to carry out the never-ending tasks of managing their diabetes every day. The trouble is that not doing what you are supposed to do only makes things worse (AKA, adolescent derangement syndrome).

Successful adaptation to diabetes has traditionally been measured by the degree to which patients achieved and maintained blood glucose and HbA1c as close to target (i.e., <7.5% in children and adolescents) as possible. Increasingly, however, optimizing quality of life has become another important measure of successful adaptation [1]. In pediatrics, it is important to remember that successful management of a chronic illness not only involves the child with the illness but the family, as well. Factors such as socioeconomic status, family structure, coping styles, the presence of maternal depression, and age can affect the family's ability to cope with diabetes and to achieve successful outcomes. In fact, increased psychological stress is directly correlated with reduced self-efficacy regarding diabetes management and with poor glucose control [2].

Professionals with expertise in the psychosocial challenges of diabetes care, such as psychologists, social workers, and nurse practitioners are essential members of the multidisciplinary diabetes care team. Regular interaction with these professionals should be encouraged and a more formal assessment should be provided for those patients and their families who exhibit psychosocial risk factors and/or have been unable to achieve diabetes care goals [3]. It is also important to involve these professionals from the time of diagnosis, as the diagnosis itself causes significant psychological distress in both the child who is diagnosed with T1D, the parents, and the family system (e.g., grandparents and other close friends and relatives). Since most children with new-onset T1D have otherwise been healthy, the diagnosis of diabetes hits parents like a ton of bricks. Providing parents with a safe place to adjust to this new chronic illness is one of the main reasons why we tend to admit all newly diagnosed children to the Children's Hospital, at least for a day or two. Of course, this has changed somewhat in association with the worldwide Covid-19 pandemic, since many families prefer to do diabetes training as outpatients to stay out of the hospital.

Common Psychosocial Challenges

Depression This is the most common psychological disorder in children and adolescents with diabetes. Numerous studies have shown that teenagers with T1D commonly have suicidal thoughts, non-adherence to the medical regimen, and psychiatric disorders that are two to three times more common than in non-diabetic teenagers. Recent data from the T1D Exchange indicate that adults with T1D who have depressive symptoms also have substantially increased HbA1c levels [4]. Research has also shown that symptoms can wax and wane throughout the course of time with diabetes, being higher in the first few years, then settling down for several years only to rise again after 10 years (Fig. 15.1) [5]. The SEARCH for Diabetes in Youth study found that rates of mild depression were 14% in youth with diabetes and that 8.6% of study participants exhibited moderate or severe symptoms [6]. Comprehensive diabetes management should include evaluation for signs of depression both informally during routine clinic visits and more formally with a standardized screening tool. Managing problems with depression will improve the quality of life and can also have an impact on glycemic control, whereas untreated

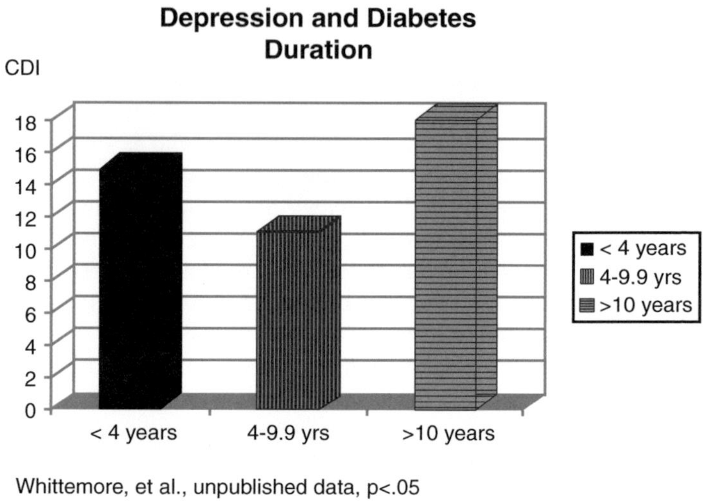

Fig. 15.1 Depression scores as a function of duration of diabetes. (From Grey et al. [5], with permission)

depression and poor glycemic control can create a vicious cycle of one negatively reinforcing the other.

Suicidality Teenagers diagnosed with T1D who experience hopelessness have been found to have increased suicidal thoughts. This illustrates the need for measurement of suicidal risk in the clinic setting, utilizing tools such as the PHQ 9 and the Columbia-Suicide Severity Rating Scale (C-SSRS), to allow for psychological intervention accompanying diabetes treatment. Suicidality with serious medical regimen non-adherence may be represent a form of passive or non-passive self-harming. Patients who identify as being hopeless toward their illness are at increased risk for suicidal ideation, as well as neglect of health care and lack of motivation to adhere to the medical regimen. Indeed, studies show that most teenagers who reported suicidal thoughts within the past year were not adherent to their medical regimen.

Disordered Eating Research indicates that disordered eating is common in both adolescent girls and boys with T1D [7]. In addition, withholding insulin is a way of purging excess calories that is unique to people with diabetes, hence the name diabulimia. This chronic state of hyperglycemia can lead to dehydration and loss of both body fat and lean muscle mass. It is reported that more than 30% of women with T1D report using insulin restriction for weight control. Patients who chronically use this method of purging are at risk for both the acute complication of diabetic ketoacidosis and more chronic complications associated with long-standing poor glycemic control. The first step in the treatment of this condition is to identify it. Warning signs can include persistently poor glycemic control, especially in combination with extreme focus on body shape and weight, strict and/or low-calorie meal plans, strict exercise regimens, and potentially repeated problems with ketonuria and/or ketoacidosis. Treatment is complex and should involve a multidisciplinary team. Initially glycemic goals should be aimed at promoting the safety of the individual as they begin to address the more complicated psychological issues, with a gradual return to more intensive glycemic targets as the individual situation warrants.

Diabetes Technologies and Distress Continuous glucose monitors (CGMs) and insulin pumps have improved dramatically over the last two decades, providing individuals with T1D many different options for self-care. Not surprisingly, some patients who use these devices may find them anxiety provoking and the volume of information can be overwhelming. Without a clear sense of how to use the data to guide treatment, the anxiety produced by CGM data can outweigh the benefits of this information. On the other hand, use of CGMs by children with T1D may be associated with a reduction in parental anxiety by decreasing the frequency of severe lows and lows at night.

Insulin pumps, which have been around for nearly 40 years, have more commonly been used than CGMs. The reasons cited for not using pumps include costs, hassles of the device, pain or discomfort with infusion site insertions, lack of trust in the technology, and a sense that the device leads the diabetes to "become visible." Nevertheless, for many patients and parents, the benefits of insulin pumps far exceed the burdens of using an insulin pump.

Anxiety In this case, anxiety is more commonly seen among parents/caregivers than by children diagnosed with diabetes, especially during the first year after diagnosis. Parents are often fearful of administering treatment as directed, and there is considerable fear around the possible development of hypoglycemia; parents of children with diabetes have a higher incidence of anxiety compared with caregivers of children without diabetes. Forty percent or more youth with diabetes also experience heightened anxiety, and the presence of anxiety worsens the prognosis of diabetes and decreases adherence with medical treatment. This is a vicious cycle where the patient concurrently requires medical and mental health treatment to break the pattern.

Interventions

Strategies to address the psychosocial implications of diabetes include family-focused interventions, behavioral contracting, stress management/coping skills, and motivational interviewing. These strategies can be utilized in one-on-one situations, peer groups, or with family systems. It cannot be stressed enough that providers with expertise in the psychosocial domain should be a part of every comprehensive diabetes team.

References

1. Whittemore R, Jaser S, Guo J, Grey M. A conceptual model of childhood adaptation to type 1 diabetes. Nurs Outlook. 2010;58:242–5.
2. Holmes CS, Chen R, Streisand R, et al. Predictors of youth diabetes care behaviors and metabolic control: a structural equation modeling approach. J Pediatr Psychol. 2006;31:770–84.

3. Delamater AM, de Wit M, McDarby V, et al. ISPAD Clinical Practice Consensus Guidelines 2014. Psychological care of children and adolescents with type 1 diabetes. Pediatr Diabetes. 2014;15(Suppl 20):232–44.
4. Trief PM, Xing D, Foster NC, et al. Depression in adults in the T1D Exchange Clinic Registry. Diabetes Care. 2014;37:1563–72.
5. Grey M, Wittemore R, Tamborlane W. Depression in type 1 diabetes in children: natural history and correlates. J Psychosom Res. 2002;53:907–11.
6. Lawrence JM, Standiford DA, Loots B, et al. Prevalence and correlates of depressed mood among youth with diabetes: the SEARCH for Diabetes in Youth study. Pediatrics. 2006;117:1348–58.
7. Doyle EA, Quinn S, Ambrosino J, Weyman K, Tamborlane WV, Jastreboff A. Disordered eating behaviors in emerging adults with type 1 diabetes: not just a female problem. J Pediatr Health Care. 2017;31:327–33.

16 Managing Type 1 Diabetes: A Young Patient's View

Patrick McAllister and Kathryn Nagel

Patrick's Story

Diagnosis

Since there are many different and unique situations that people with T1D must navigate through during their lives, it might be helpful to highlight some of the most prominent ones. This first event – diagnosis – is one that every individual with T1D must go through, and is also arguably the toughest event to overcome. My diagnosis came as a complete surprise, as my pediatrician found large ketones in my urine during a routine checkup despite my complete lack of symptoms. Unlike many others, I did not have to deal with a brutal period of relentless thirst and urination accompanied by severe weight loss, fatigue, and utter confusion.

Despite an absence of diabetes-related symptoms, the realization that I had diabetes was overwhelming. My lasting memory was sitting in a hospital bed watching my mother cry and my father hold back tears. I had never seen both like this and I had no sense of what my life would become. When an adolescent patient (or any patient for that matter) is diagnosed with T1D, it is crucial

P. McAllister (✉)
University of Connecticut, School of Medicine, Farmington, CT, USA

K. Nagel
Yale New Haven Hospital, Internal Medicine/Pediatrics Residency, New Haven, CT, USA

W. V. Tamborlane (ed.), *Diabetes in Children and Adolescents*, Contemporary Endocrinology,
https://doi.org/10.1007/978-3-030-64133-7_16

that someone lays the groundwork for what T1D truly is. Obviously, the Instructional Manual (see Chap. 20) comes with standard sections like, *"What is T1D," "What is insulin,"* and *"How do I count carbs",* but there are a few additional topics that are sometimes left out. Nevertheless, these omissions can make all the difference in how your newly diagnosed adolescent comprehends and compensates for having T1D.

I also remember that one of my doctors said something that completely changed my outlook on what T1D was. "Being diagnosed with T1D is not a death sentence, not this terribly damning disease that is going to ruin your life, but rather a lifestyle change," he said. He stressed that the diagnosis of T1D did not stop you from doing anything you want to do in life. Teens who could cope with the day-to-day challenges of T1D would eventually succeed in self-management of diabetes, as well as whatever else they wish to accomplish in life. It also helps to remind them that people like Nick Jonas, Halle Barry, and Sonia Sotomayor all live and thrive with T1D. T1D will not stop you from becoming a better singer, actress, or judge if that is something you want to be.

It is very important to reassure your patients that they are not alone when it comes to their T1D. In fact, managing T1D for any newly diagnosed patient requires a community effort that includes family members, friends, teachers, doctors, nurses, nutritionists, and therapists, to name a few. Even with these helping hands, there exists a void for newly diagnosed teens with T1D, when it comes to having someone with whom you can relate and connect with. I was very fortunate that both my older cousin and one of my best friends also had T1D. I knew I could reach out to either of them any time I needed anything. On the other hand, I know people with T1D who went years before meeting and conversing with another individual with T1D. While it may sound of secondary importance, helping your patients connect with others in the T1D community can make the world of difference in their acceptance of their new lifestyle. Social media and other online communities such as Beyond Type 1 and JDRF are great initial resources for kids and teens with T1D. Summer Diabetes Camp also provides opportunities to meet other teens with T1D, and the College Diabetes Network provides a platform that helps newly diagnosed patients meet and connect with people of similar age. The resources are out there, and providing these outlets to your patients will show them that you care more than just about their ability to prick their fingers and give themselves the correct dose of insulin. [*Doctor's note: in the 1990's, going to Diabetes Camp in the summer was where many youngsters with T1D first discovered an interest in trying to use an insulin pump*]

Eventually, all your patients will have to leave the hospital and return home. Indeed, at Yale, they do not keep you more than 2 or 3 days in the hospital. The first few weeks at home were some of the scariest times I have ever had with my T1D. When I was in the hospital, I did not have to religiously count carbs or give myself insulin because it was mostly done for me. But when I got home, I had to measure how much cereal I had for breakfast and repeatedly prick my finger to measure blood glucose levels. Of course, this made me realize how drastic a lifestyle-change this disease was going to be. All the resources in the world could not have prevented me from feeling frightened, overwhelmed, and alone during this time period.

My take-home message is that diabetes providers need to be mindful of how delicate the first couple weeks can be for their adolescent patients. In addition, be mindful that your teen patients will be grappling with teenage hormone surges, middle and high school dramas, challenging course work, sports, and countless other hurdles. Adding T1D to this equation is enough to make anyone's head spin! Reassuring your patients and their families that these feelings are normal can give everyone peace of mind during this immensely challenging period. The good news is that things start to settle down during the first 3–4 months of having diabetes.

Provider Visits

I would thank any god or deity if I never have to relive my first weeks of having T1D. This section, however, is even more vital because it pertains to events that will happen for the rest of your patients' lives, namely, the dreaded *doctor appointments*. Visiting a provider, whether it be a pediatric endocrinologist, nurse practitioner, nutritionist, therapist, or even school counselor comes with its own set of challenges; challenges that are even more difficult by simply being a teenager. One of my doctor's calls this "adolescent derangement syndrome." He says that it is not unusual for teenagers to assume that T1D will go away, if they just ignore it. Unfortunately, that only makes things worse.

It is no surprise that when I was a teenager I had a love-hate relationship with my endocrinology appointments. On the one hand, I was fortunate enough to be blessed with an incredible T1D team from the nurses all the way up to the doctors. Everyone was friendly and seemed to take an interest in my life, even the stuff that had nothing to do with T1D. When my provider started every appointment with a couple questions about how my life was going (e.g., school, sports, and band), it allowed me to open up and made me feel that this appointment was more than just a data point on my HbA1c graph. I understand that it might be difficult for you to openly converse with some of your adolescent patients, but for me, beginning every T1D appointment with something other than T1D seemed to help. The other good news about one of my clinic appointments was that I sold my doctor a whole year of tickets for the town's High School sports teams. It was only later that I discovered that he never went to any of the games.

The part of my appointments that I dreaded the most was the point-of-care measurements of HbA1c level in the clinic. As someone who had a 3.98 GPA in high school and a 3.99 GPA in college, I hated getting bad grades; they make me feel inadequate and incompetent. Having said this, it is relatively easy to get a good grade on a test if you pay attention in class, study in advance, and get enough sleep the night before the exam. On the other hand, you can try your absolute hardest to get a "good grade" on you HbA1c test and still not get the results you want.

Three months is a long period of time to cram into a single quantitative evaluation, and I vividly remember countless occasions sitting in the doctor's office with thoughts racing through my head while I waited for the results of my HbA1c: *Were my glucose numbers too high? Should I have tried to change my insulin doses? Why couldn't I get my glucose levels below 200,*

4 weeks ago? Why can't I just manage my T1D better. I became increasingly negative and blamed myself for my T1D shortcomings. Fortunately, at each visit, I would bet a dollar with one of my doctors that my HbA1c was higher or lower than a certain level (in professional football betting this is called an over/under bet). I quickly realized that he picked a cut-off level that was always higher than actual HbA1c value that was measured that day. It made both of us feel good, even though I won the dollar every time by betting low.

"There's no such thing as a bad blood sugar level." I was not aware of this philosophy until I was talking with a pediatric psychiatrist 9 years into my life with T1D. I just assumed that if your blood glucose level was between 70 and 180 mg/dL, it was a "good" number, while anything outside that range was a "bad" number; in range = good, outside range = bad. The problem with this philosophy is that it becomes too overbearing to handle, especially for a teenager or young adult who is in constant pursuit of gratification from every corner of his/her life. Sometimes glucose levels spike or drop for reasons unknown to anyone, and to chalk those irregularities up to a "failure" on the patient's behalf is unfair. While some glucose and HbA1c levels may be "in range" (i.e., good), others may be "out of range" (i.e., bad). However, that does not mean that you are good or bad. In fact, every number is a data point of information that can be used to better future T1D management.

If this way of viewing blood glucose and HbA1C levels was provided to me as a teenager, I would have undoubtedly felt less stressed about feeling that every second of every day I needed to have my levels in range. Impressing onto your adolescent patients that they are not to blame for what is happening to them, but rather that you and your patients will work together to regulate glucose levels will ease the incredible burden that they unquestionably feel every day. It would also be helpful to teach them that insulin requirements are almost always increasing during adolescence and you can tell when you need to increase insulin doses when your sugar levels are too high. Once you get into your 20's, the opposite may be true – you have to start reducing some of your insulin doses.

Doctors and other practitioners should also know that we are constantly trying to make life easier, even in minor ways. We constantly think about our T1D and how it might be improved. However, many times at my doctor's appointments, I was too shy or scared to ask questions about my T1D management. For this reason, I urge you to pick and prod your patients and gather their questions and concerns about their own care because some trends might not show up in insulin pump or continuous glucose monitor (CGM) data. Additionally, I always loved when my endocrinologists explained concepts to help me better understand my T1D care or introduced a new insulin pump or CGM that I might want to try. Exploring different options with your patients and including them in the decisions will open up doors to potential better regimens, as well as give them a sense of empowerment that they have control over their T1D.

Taboo Topics

I thought it would be wise to include this section in our "A Teenager's View" chapter because despite flying under the radar many times in healthcare conversations, all of these "taboo topics" are a part of teenage life. These situations can be extremely challenging to navigate blindly and most teenagers are reluctant to initiate any sort of dialogue about them with their healthcare providers. Nevertheless, they are integral for all individuals with T1D to understand and become comfortable with, as a lack of knowledge in these areas can be dangerous.

I will begin by pointing out that it will be nearly impossible for you to have a proper two-way conversation with your adolescent patients about sensitive topics if their moms and dads are also in the room. I can recount times when I "held things back" at the doctor's office because I did not want to have to admit to anything in front of my parents. Creating a safe, open, and confidential environment is paramount to the success of these discussions. The best way is to ask your patient's parents/guardians to give you and your patient some privacy. Likewise, assure your patients that nothing divulged between the two of you will be shared with anyone. That goes a long way for easing tensions about the possibility of anything leaking out and reaching unwanted ears.

First up on our list of taboo topics is sex. Even if someone has already had the "birds and the bees" talk with your teenage patients prior to your appointments, I highly doubt the version they were taught included the fact that the birds and bees might have T1D. As a teenager, I never had the sex conversation with my endocrinologist or any healthcare provider for that matter. Consequently, I had to learn everything by trial and error. When I started having sex, I noticed having frequent low sugar levels during intercourse. These hypoglycemic episodes were almost always accompanied by erectile dysfunction and I could not perform until those low sugar levels were corrected (which usually took anywhere from 15 to 30 minutes). I understood that sex was a physical activity, which made me more prone to hypoglycemia, but this was hard to explain to my partner. It was not until years later when I was having a conversation with one of my friends with T1D about this very topic that he exclaimed, "I know! That happens to me too. It's the worst!" If this topic comes up with one of your young adult patients, male or female, help them understand that erectile dysfunction and loss of libido can happen with low glucose levels. At the very least, it will give them reassurance that it is not their fault that they are having trouble performing. Furthermore, creating a plan for how to prevent these problems, such as having a snack beforehand, can provide your young adult T1D patients with both comfort and encouragement when it comes to sex.

A much more common problem in the teenagers with T1D is the use of recreational drugs; especially, alcohol and marijuana. I personally do not have experience with any other recreational drugs and frankly do not condone their use under any circumstances. However, if one of your patients is frequently using one of these drugs (e.g., cocaine, LSD, and heroin), I am sorry to say that T1D is the least of his/her problems. On the other hand, having a conversation with your teen patients on how marijuana and/or alcohol will affect their T1D management is extremely important. With respect to marijuana, an overall lack of drive to properly manage one's T1D proves much more troublesome than any effects from the marijuana itself. Alcohol on the other hand, is a completely different animal. Since alcohol lowers glucose levels by suppressing the liver's breakdown of stored glycogen, drinking alcohol can be very dangerous for individuals with T1D. Combine a tendency to hypoglycemia with a drug that exaggerates the risk for hypoglycemia and a dangerous situation can become lethal. There have been times when drinking that I honestly could not tell if I was drunk or low and had to refer to my CGM in order to tell. Since this is such an acutely threatening situation, explain the physiology to your teen and young adult patients and urge them to take measures to ensure their safety while drinking.

Another important note to keep in mind is that when teens and young adults are participating in recreational use of alcohol and/or marijuana, the scenario almost always involves a party culture. Teens want to appear cool to their friends, significant others, and anyone around them while partying. The "I can hang with the cool kids" mentality is especially dangerous for adolescents and young adults with T1D because they often neglect their T1D care while trying to maintain this facade. I remember feeling this pressure in high school and college, like it was uncool to check my blood glucose levels or take my insulin. Be mindful of this and use strategies and routines to try to help them see past this irresponsible and risky philosophy of thought. Emphasize to them that their T1D does not need to prevent them from having a good time, but their health should always come first.

In college, I set up what I called "safety nets" for myself when I used to go out and party. I made sure at least one other person at the party knew I had T1D, and likewise what to do should I start acting funky. I also often refrained from heavy bolusing during parties so that I knew I would not go low and risk a severe hypoglycemic episode. If you talk in a down-to-earth manner with your teen and young adult patients about these topics, and work together to create proactive and practical plans for their T1D care, you will give these patients a sense of security and assurance that they do not have to choose between either sex, drinking, and partying or their T1D. When in college, you should also tell your roommate that you have T1D and what they should do if you get hypoglycemic, especially after partying.

Kathryn's Story

My name is Kathryn Nagel, and I am currently a resident physician finishing my last year of combined residency in Internal Medicine and Pediatrics (Med/Peds) at Yale. Long before I was a doctor, I was a patient. I was diagnosed with type 1 diabetes when I was 18 months old. Below is my story, which has greatly influenced my path as a doctor, and, I hope, will be helpful for you too.

Early Life with T1D

People always start their T1D story with their diagnosis. For better or worse, I do not actually recall my diagnosis, since it occurred when I was 18 months old. I have heard plenty about it from my parents, who still recall the trauma even now almost 30 years later. For them, this was an earth-shattering event from which everything would change. Someone during that initial hospitalization had told them that I would never live a normal life, and that most likely by the time I was a teenager and young adult, I would be quite sick. My parents lived with this fear throughout my childhood.

As a result, I grew up with a deep determination to prove whoever said that was wrong. In many ways, I count it as a blessing that I was diagnosed so young. For me, the only thing I knew was life with T1D. I was able to test my blood sugar before I even knew how to read two-digit numbers. I learned that feeling sweaty meant I might be low. Taking insulin before meals was as routine as brushing teeth and setting the table. I never grew angry at my disease or at what was being asked of me, because for me it was just how life was.

I was also extremely lucky to have the parents I had and their support. They understood the magnitude of a disease like this and taught me the careful balance of self-acceptance and forgiveness without self-pity. There was no such thing as a "bad" number in our house, just an opportunity to problem solve when things were not in range. I was taught to be part of this problem solving from a very young age. From choosing my shot sites to eventually dosing my insulin, my parents always encouraged me to be part of the care and take over actions as soon as it was developmentally appropriate, always providing support along the way. Bottom line, I was raised with a can-do attitude, which I believe greatly affected my later years of life with the disease.

Childhood

As a kid, our family's goal was twofold: keep the A1c levels in range and live a normal life. Diabetes was taken seriously, but participating in all the normal activities of childhood was taken just as seriously. I was taught that kids with diabetes could do anything other kids could do, they just always had to be more prepared. I was lucky to have a rich and fulfilling childhood. I played soccer, had sleepovers, went on school trips, and travelled with my family.

Diabetes had to be respected in all activities (e.g., test your blood sugar before a soccer game, always carry juice, bring a doctor's note while travelling, and bring extras of all supplies), but never let it get in the way. More importantly, it was *never* accepted to use diabetes as an excuse to not do something. If I had a low blood sugar and had to sit out for a few minutes then that was what needed to happen, but it was instilled in me deeply to never use diabetes as an excuse. This discipline served me well when I got older.

One source of conflict I often had with my parents and providers was over control, especially of little things, namely, things that seemed small to them were huge to me. My doctors always wanted me to use more sites for my shots, but I was insistent on only using my arms and legs. We ultimately compromised and I was not forced to use sites I did not want to, but encouraged to rotate around the sites I was comfortable with. I have since worked with many children, and found similar stubbornness. Things that might seem small to adults, such as injecting yourself in the stomach, can be huge to a kid. It is important to recognize how big those choices can be to someone that age, and engage them in the discussion, giving them control wherever it can reasonably be done.

Perhaps the largest source of conflict with my family and medical team was my insistence on not transitioning to pump therapy. When I was diagnosed, there were no modern pumps or continuous glucose monitors. In fact, Humalog and Lantus did not even exist back then. I used NPH and Regular drawn up in a syringe and vial and tested my blood sugar with a meter that took 2 minutes to get a single reading. As new insulins and technologies came out, I tried them, but there was one change I was unwilling to make: transitioning to an insulin pump.

Starting when I was about 10 years old, my medical providers kept trying to convince me to go on a pump. They said that once I got used to it I would love it. My parents, however, who knew my personality, understood it would be damaging to make such an important decision about my care against my will. Instead they made a deal with me: If I kept my A1c in range no one would give me a hard time about the method of care I chose to use. If my A1c went out of range we would reopen the discussion. The empowerment and trust they showed in me proved incredibly important as I reached my adolescent years and developed my own identity as a young person with T1D.

Adolescence

Adolescence is a time for individuation and identity formation. T1D inherently creates major challenges in this process. In fact, I would argue that some of the requirements of T1D are exactly counter to the developmental requirements of this age group. Young people with diabetes are taught that they are dependent on their parents and doctors, and forced to share a large amount of personal information with them. This is not consistent with the individuation that is supposed to happen during adolescence. The sharing of all your numbers and intimate details of your daily life with doctors and parents can feel deeply violating. Adolescents, especially young women, are already prone to feeling self-conscious and the every 3-month "report card" feel of the A1c does not help.

I was fiercely independent as a teenager, probably more than the average teen. It was a point of pride for me that the high school nurse did not know my name. Though I may have been extreme, I think the feeling of intrusion I experienced with the scrutiny over my numbers and performance is a fairly universal experience. I left many doctors' appointments in tears. I remember being particularly reactive to being talked down to. I had been managing this disease for many years and I was an expert on it, just as I was an expert on my own body.

I do not think there is any way to live with T1D and not be an expert on the disease. As a provider, I always try to recognize this fact and honor the experience of my young patients. While there are many areas where they likely need help, the truth is they have a lot to teach us about their own experience. I was much more likely to open up to and trust a provider who treated me with respect than one who talked to me like a little kid.

Though I am not sure the adults in my life realized it, I experienced a lot of fear and anxiety during those tumultuous years. It was hard to navigate and though I would have *never* admitted any emotions that expressed vulnerability, I felt very vulnerable.

I often marvel at how much easier it is to control my diabetes now than it was then. Some of this is just the chaos of teenage life – but honestly, speaking as someone who is currently a medical resident working crazy hours, I think a lot of it was just hormones. They can REALLY affect your blood sugar.

After high school, I spent some time working at a diabetes camp for girls. I was the counselor in a cabin of 15-year-old girls. Similar to my experience, their concerns did not always align with their doctors and their parents. Complications were a distant concept, not really dwelt on. A1cs mattered more in the judgment given by others, less in what they implied for your future health. Occupying a lot of brain space was how diabetes would affect your interactions with peers – dating, hooking up (what do you do with pump tubing?), drinking alcohol, etc. Moreover, how do you develop self-esteem when you often feel a sense of failure trying to manage such a tough disease?

Like me, these girls would hide their vulnerabilities at all costs, often by acting like they did not care. Young people need support, and while a huge portion of that support comes from parents and healthcare professionals, they also need it from peers. Helping these young people have enough self-respect to be able to share the details of their condition with their friends and potential romantic partners is one of the greatest services we can give them.

The most important thing that I developed during this time was a positive sense of who I was with diabetes. I felt no need to hide it, which allowed me to get the support I needed once I left my home for college. If there is one thing healthcare providers should focus on for teenagers is that they should develop a positive sense of self and a positive relationship with diabetes, no matter how hard and frustrating it is.

Young Adulthood

Turning 18 and finally being deemed independent was very exciting for me. As someone who always wanted to have autonomy, I loved being able to go to doctors' appointments by myself. Of course, there were many things that were challenging about this time. I think the hardest part was learning how to navigate insurance and order my own supplies. I had not realized how complicated that was. I know my parents were very nervous about me going off to college with diabetes. I felt less so, but it was still scary. They bought me a Dexcom continuous glucose monitor, which would wake me up at night if I were low. I, of course, did not always wear it (I found the thing annoying), but I realized that my parents were afraid of a low blood sugar in the middle of the night that could be very serious, especially because they were not there to help.

What became critical to my success as a young adult was my network of very supportive friends. I was not shy at all about my diagnosis, so everyone who knew me knew I had it. While there were plenty of people who were ignorant about the disease, I was happy to teach them about it and my close friends were my biggest supporters. As we started experimenting with alcohol, they made it a game to check my blood sugar level and sometimes we would guess and check theirs too. I felt that I was not alone with the disease and if anything ever went wrong, there were a lot of people around me who knew what to do and how to help.

As many young people do, I stayed with my pediatric endocrine team until I was 22. Transitioning to an adult provider was hard, since my initial doctor and I did not click. He made me so angry my blood pressure spiked, to which he suggested putting me on a blood pressure medication. He did not know much about me and did not seem interested in connecting with me as a person, so I had no trust in him and was not inclined to listen to anything he had to say.

I subsequently learned that transitioning to adult care can be smoothed by a trusting relationship with your provider and that building a therapeutic alliance is essential. As a young person, it is easy to convince yourself that you are fine and disappear from care, as long as someone will keep prescribing your insulin and supplies. This is a real shame because it really is helpful to have a healthcare team on your side helping you navigate your way through early adulthood. I ultimately found a doctor who understood my personality. She never told me what to do, explored my struggles, and was willing to have open conversations about options for care. She guided me through trying insulin pump therapy on my own terms and supported my need to make my own decisions.

For every young person with diabetes, there can be a disconnect between what doctors and parents think is important and what the young person thinks is important. For me, it was much more important to be able to live a normal life than to live the perfect lifestyle and achieve perfect glucose and HbA1c numbers. Having a doctor who understood this and did not judge me was critical. While it is important to make sure young people know the consequences of their actions, it is also important to recognize where they are developmentally. As during my childhood, it was essential that diabetes should not prevent me from living like my peers. I was not willing to say, “Oh I’m diabetic, I can’t do that.” This mindset kept me from developing resentment towards my disease, which I firmly believe has been a huge part of my success in living with it.

For me, one of the most valuable things I did during my young adult years was getting involved with other groups of young people with diabetes. I was lucky enough to find passionate groups of peers who turned out to be great friends and an understanding support network. Our advocacy furthered our feeling of empowerment and made living as a young person with diabetes a lot easier. While advocacy is not for everyone, I think the connection with other people going through similar experiences can be super helpful. As a provider, the worst outcomes I have seen in young adults with diabetes come from trying to do things completely alone. Young adulthood is a tumultuous time, but with a trusting healthcare team and supportive friends, the bumps in the road can be navigated successfully and smoothly.

To the Providers Who Serve Young People with T1D

Thank you for caring about and serving this most special of groups. If I were to give one piece of advice, it would be this: there is no formula or technology that can fix this disease. Perfect numbers will not be had with even the highest tech pump, CGM, fast-acting insulin, and smart basal. These things can and will help, but the truth is that even a good old vial and syringe can do the trick. The solution lies in the patient, and the most powerful thing we can do for our patients as providers is empower them to take ownership of their disease and its management. Technologies and new insulins can unquestionably be helpful, and the support of providers is critical, but even the best technologies and most caring providers cannot take away the burden of this disease.

Instead of greeting patients by scouring through pages and pages of data, chat with them. Know them as people. Help them know themselves, and teach them to honor themselves. What it takes to manage this disease is so impressive. If we can help young people realize their potential and feel pride in themselves and all they've accomplished, we've done them a great service.

Conclusion

It is important to note that Patrick indicated that daily life with T1D has its ups and downs. He would contend that every person with T1D, regardless of age, has those days when you feel like you are falling apart; like the world is crashing down around you and that there is nothing you can do about it; days when your blood glucose levels will not stay in range no matter how hard you try. On the other hand, virtually all of Kathryn's life has been affected by management of her diabetes. Nevertheless, her message was that diabetes need not interfere with being successful in whatever task you undertake. As a healthcare provider, a take-home message from both is to listen to and understand the challenges that your patients face every day. Demonstrating to your patients that they are in control and are not alone will give them the comfort they need to be receptive to your advice and the confidence to manage this whirlwind of a life with T1D.

Part II

Type 2 Diabetes

Nonalcoholic Fatty Liver Disease (NAFLD) Association with Pediatric Diabetes

17

Nicola Santoro, Rachel Goldberg-Gel, and Sonia Caprio

Nonalcoholic Fatty Liver Disease (NAFLD) in Pediatrics

Nonalcoholic fatty liver disease (NAFLD) is the most common complication of obesity and the most common liver disease occurring in children [1]. The prevalence of NAFLD in pediatrics has been estimated to be about 3–8% with a peak of 35–50% among obese youth [1–3]. The prevalence of NAFLD is associated with both male gender and ethnicity, as Hispanic youth show the highest risk for developing NAFLD, while African Americans seem to be protected even in the presence of severe obesity and insulin resistance [3, 4]. NAFLD describes a wide spectrum of disease severity from simple intrahepatic fat accumulation (steatosis) to non-alcoholic steatohepatitis (NASH), cirrhosis, and hepatocellular carcinoma (HCC) [3, 5].

The long-term consequences of early onset NAFLD are poorly understood because of the paucity of prospective studies [6, 7]. One retrospective study by Feldstein and colleagues has shown

N. Santoro (✉) · R. Goldberg-Gel · S. Caprio
Yale-New Haven Children's Hospital, Department of Pediatrics, Yale School of Medicine, New Haven, CT, USA
e-mail: nicola.santoro@yale.edu

W. V. Tamborlane (ed.), *Diabetes in Children and Adolescents*, Contemporary Endocrinology,
https://doi.org/10.1007/978-3-030-64133-7_17

that onset of NAFLD during puberty is associated with high risk of end-stage liver disease during the second decade of life [6]. Despite being such a common disease, the precise mechanisms leading to NAFLD are still largely unknown. However, intrahepatic fat accumulation appears to be driven by at least three major mechanisms: (1) adipose tissue lipolysis that accounts for ~60% of free fatty acids (FFA) in the liver, (2) hepatic de novo lipogenesis – the mechanism responsible for the conversion of carbohydrates into lipids that accounts for ~25% of intrahepatic fat, and (3) dietary lipids that contribute ~15% to intrahepatic fat [8]. The imbalance among these three sources of fatty acids for the liver probably play a major in the development of NAFLD in the context of type 1 and type 2 diabetes.

NAFLD in Obesity, Insulin Resistance, and Type 2 Diabetes (T2D)

Studies in children and adolescents have shown that the consequences of NAFLD extend beyond the liver. D'Adamo et al. have shown that intrahepatic fat content per se – independent of visceral fat, intramuscular fat, age, gender, and BMI – is a major determinant of hepatic, adipose, and muscle insulin resistance predisposing obese youth to prediabetes and T2D [9]. Data provided by the NASH CRN [10], a consortium study of NAFLD and NASH in children and adults, have shown that higher levels of intrahepatic fat content and inflammation in youth with NAFLD are associated with increased susceptibility to prediabetes and T2D [11]. In particular, it has been shown that girls with NAFLD had approximately 1.6-fold higher odds of prediabetes and five-fold higher odds of T2D as compared to boys [11]. Nonalcoholic steatohepatitis (NASH) tends to be more prevalent among youth with T2D (43.2%) than in those with normal glucose tolerance (22%) [11]. Similarly, youth with prediabetes and T2D have an increased risk of steatohepatitis than with obese youth with normal glucose tolerance [11].

While the mechanisms linking NAFLD to T2D are unclear, it is possible that intrahepatic accumulation of free fatty acids

(FFAs) results in an overproduction of diacylglycerol (DAG) and ceramides species, which in turn affect insulin signaling in the liver causing increased hepatic glucose production [12, 13]. The overall effect of the metabolic changes occurring in youth with NAFLD is to exacerbate the degree of insulin resistance naturally occurring during puberty leading to prediabetes and T2D [14].

Whether NAFLD is a cause or a consequence of insulin resistance remains unclear. Recently, Trico et al. studied 73 obese youth with fatty liver and followed them for 2 years [15]. After 2 years, about 25% of participants had developed NAFLD. It is particularly noteworthy that those who developed NAFLD had a more severe degree of insulin resistance at baseline [15]. This study, although small, suggests that insulin resistance may be the pillar on which NAFLD is built. However, it is likely that FFAs, accumulating in the liver in amounts that exceed the ability of the liver to remove them, also contribute. Consequently, compounds such as DAG and ceramides are produced that worsen insulin resistance, thereby creating a vicious circle that is difficult to break.

NAFLD and T1D

Information regarding the association between T1D and fatty liver is sparse and controversial. Studies in adults and children have suggested that an association between these two conditions might exist, but the pathogenic underpinnings remain unclear. In one study of 106 children with T1D aged 8 months to 15 years, fatty liver was detected in 11.3% of patients and the presence of fatty liver correlated with poorer glycemic control when compared to patients without detectable fatty liver [16]. Compared to adults with T1D, the prevalence of fatty liver tends to be higher than in children, ranging from 24% [17] to 50.2% [18, 19]. Interestingly, in a recent study of newly diagnosed Chinese patients with diabetes, participants with ketosis at diagnosis had significantly higher fatty liver prevalence (61.8%) as compared to those with long-standing well-controlled T1D patients (15.4%) [20]. The problem with some of these studies is that in many cases ultrasound, which is not considered a strong technique to detect NAFLD, was used to detect fatty liver, and the effect of obesity was not always considered. One recent retrospective study of patients with diabetes who had undergone liver biopsy reported a similar risk of developing steatosis and cirrhosis among patients with T1D and T2D who were matched for potential confounders including sex, age, and obesity status [21].

More recently, studies assessing liver fat content using magnetic resonance imaging (MRI) have shown that the prevalence of fatty liver in adults with T1D is about 9% [22]. Two studies in adults with T1D found lower hepatic fat content in subjects with T1D compared to controls [23, 24]. Interestingly, studies using MRI, a robust technique to detect intrahepatic fat, tended to show a lower prevalence of NAFLD in subjects with T1D than in controls [23, 24]. The reason for these differences is unclear, but one possibility is that exogenous insulin efficiently blocks adipose tissue lipolysis and FFA flux from adipose tissue to the liver, particularly in patients with optimal glycemic control. Adipose tissue lipolysis is, indeed, probably the main source of FFA to the liver in non-obese individuals. Despite evidence for this potential mechanism, prospective studies designed to characterize more fully the physiopathology of NAFLD in youth with T1D are needed, as many questions about the relationship between these two diseases remain unanswered.

Therapeutic Approach to NAFLD

Since there are no currently approved pharmacological treatments for NAFLD, the main treatments are represented by implementing changes in lifestyle, such as encouraging healthy dietary changes and weight loss. Recent data in children and adolescents suggest that dietary added sugars and some dietary fatty acids favor the onset and progression of NAFLD. Therefore, recent dietary interventions have focused on reducing or eliminating these components from the diet. In a recent 8-week open-label, randomized clinical trial, Schwimmer JB et al. have shown that an intervention characterized by limiting free sugar intake to <3% of daily calorie intake reduces intrahepatic fat content measured by MRI by ~25% and ALT by ~40% [25]. Another study in which the investigators manipulated the composition of fatty acids by increasing the amount of omega-3 polyunsaturated fatty acids (PUFA) and reducing the omega-6 PUFA in the diet of obese adolescents with MRI-proven NAFLD showed a 25% decrease of the intrahepatic fat content over 12 weeks and an improvement of insulin resistance and lipid profiles [26].

Along with dietary intervention, several drugs have been tested in adults and youth with NAFLD. In 2011, Lavine J et al. tested metformin and vitamin E against placebo in a group of youth with biopsy-proven NASH [27]. This was a 96-week study and the primary outcome was the reduction of the ALT of more than 50% compared to the baseline values. Although a higher proportion of subjects taking metformin and vitamin E showed a greater improvement of histological features at the end of the study compared to placebo (28%), these differences were not statistically significant [27]. More recently, investigators from the NASH-CRN consortium tested the effect of cysteamine bitartrate delayed release (CBDR) versus placebo on fatty liver in youth. The primary outcome was the improvement of liver histology over 52 weeks. At the end of the study, there was no difference in liver histology between the group treated with CBDR (28%) and that treated with placebo (22%) [28]. Therefore, to date none of the clinical trials testing drugs for the treatment of NAFLD in youth have been successful.

More encouraging are data from studies in adults. Recent investigations have been focused on the role of anti-diabetic drugs as a therapy for fatty liver disease. Seminal work by Kenneth Cusi has shown that pioglitazone is effective in reducing intrahepatic fat content and improving liver histology in adult patients with impaired glucose tolerance or diabetes and NAFLD [29].

More recent studies in adults have focused on the effect of GLP-1 analogs and SGLT2 inhibitors on NAFLD. In a double-blinded placebo-controlled trial, Armstrong et al. showed that a 48-week treatment with liraglutide was superior to placebo in determining resolution of NAFLD in patients with diabetes [30].

As expected, the group of patients taking liraglutide also experienced significant weight loss over the course of the intervention. Other studies [31] have shown that treatment with GLP-1 analogs produced a significant improvement of the liver, including liver fibrosis, which is a worrisome feature of NAFLD, as it is a prelude to cirrhosis of the liver.

The use of SGLT2 inhibitors as therapeutic agents for NAFLD is more recent. Erikson et al. have shown that treatment with dapagliflozin causes an 18% reduction of intrahepatic content after 12 weeks treatment in patients with T2D and NAFLD [32]. Similarly, Kuchay et al. showed that empagliflozin is superior to the standard treatment (glucose lowering drugs and dietary recommendations) in improving intrahepatic fat content in patients with T2D [33].

While these studies have provided very encouraging data, the main problem is that the NAFLD phenotype reappears as soon as the intervention is discontinued. Nevertheless, these interventions might be used in the future to reduce the degree of NAFLD, but not as a cure. Moreover, none of the anti-diabetic drugs tested in adults have ever been tested in a pediatric population. The latter represents a major gap in knowledge that needs to be addressed to provide an effective treatment to the ever-growing number of youth who develop NAFLD early in life.

References

1. Goldner D, Lavine JE. Nonalcoholic fatty liver disease in children: unique considerations and challenges. Gastroenterology. 2020. https://doi.org/10.1053/j.gastro.2020.01.048.
2. Schwimmer JB, et al. Obesity, insulin resistance, and other clinicopathological correlates of pediatric nonalcoholic fatty liver disease. J Pediatr. 2003;143:500–5. https://doi.org/10.1067/s0022-3476(03)00325-1.
3. Schwimmer JB, McGreal N, Deutsch R, Finegold MJ, Lavine JE. Influence of gender, race, and ethnicity on suspected fatty liver in obese adolescents. Pediatrics. 2005;115:e561–5. https://doi.org/10.1542/peds.2004-1832.
4. Browning JD, et al. Prevalence of hepatic steatosis in an urban population in the United States: impact of ethnicity. Hepatology. 2004;40:1387–95. https://doi.org/10.1002/hep.20466.

5. Angulo P. Nonalcoholic fatty liver disease. N Engl J Med. 2002;346:1221–31. https://doi.org/10.1056/NEJMra011775.
6. Feldstein AE, et al. The natural history of non-alcoholic fatty liver disease in children: a follow-up study for up to 20 years. Gut. 2009;58:1538–44. https://doi.org/10.1136/gut.2008.171280.
7. Adams LA, et al. The natural history of nonalcoholic fatty liver disease: a population-based cohort study. Gastroenterology. 2005;129:113–21. https://doi.org/10.1053/j.gastro.2005.04.014.
8. Donnelly KL, et al. Sources of fatty acids stored in liver and secreted via lipoproteins in patients with nonalcoholic fatty liver disease. J Clin Invest. 2005;115:1343–51. https://doi.org/10.1172/jci23621.
9. D'Adamo E, et al. Central role of fatty liver in the pathogenesis of insulin resistance in obese adolescents. Diabetes Care. 2010;33:1817–22. https://doi.org/10.2337/dc10-0284.
10. Lavine JE, Schwimmer JB. Pediatric initiatives within the Nonalcoholic Steatohepatitis-Clinical Research Network (NASH CNR). J Pediatr Gastroenterol Nutr. 2003;37:220–1. https://doi.org/10.1097/00005176-200309000-00002.
11. Newton KP, et al. Prevalence of prediabetes and type 2 diabetes in children with nonalcoholic fatty liver disease. JAMA Pediatr. 2016;170:e161971. https://doi.org/10.1001/jamapediatrics.2016.1971.
12. Samuel VT, Shulman GI. Nonalcoholic fatty liver disease, insulin resistance, and ceramides. N Engl J Med. 2019;381:1866–9. https://doi.org/10.1056/NEJMcibr1910023.
13. Kusminski CM, Scherer PE. Lowering ceramides to overcome diabetes. Science. 2019;365:319–20. https://doi.org/10.1126/science.aax6594.
14. Amiel SA, Sherwin RS, Simonson DC, Lauritano AA, Tamborlane WV. Impaired insulin action in puberty. A contributing factor to poor glycemic control in adolescents with diabetes. N Engl J Med. 1986;315:215–9. https://doi.org/10.1056/nejm198607243150402.
15. Trico D, et al. Metabolic features of nonalcoholic fatty liver (NAFL) in obese adolescents: findings from a multiethnic cohort. Hepatology. 2018;68:1376–90. https://doi.org/10.1002/hep.30035.
16. Al-Hussaini AA, Sulaiman NM, Alzahrani MD, Alenizi AS, Khan M. Prevalence of hepatopathy in type 1 diabetic children. BMC Pediatr. 2012;12:160. https://doi.org/10.1186/1471-2431-12-160.
17. Gaiani S, et al. Nonalcoholic fatty liver disease (NAFLD) in nonobese patients with diabetes: prevalence and relationships with hemodynamic alterations detected with Doppler sonography(). J Ultrasound. 2009;12:1–5. https://doi.org/10.1016/j.jus.2008.12.002.
18. Targher G, et al. Prevalence of non-alcoholic fatty liver disease and its association with cardiovascular disease in patients with type 1 diabetes. J Hepatol. 2010;53:713–8. https://doi.org/10.1016/j.jhep.2010.04.030.
19. Targher G, et al. Nonalcoholic fatty liver disease is independently associated with an increased incidence of chronic kidney disease in patients

with type 1 diabetes. Diabetes Care. 2014;37:1729–36. https://doi.org/10.2337/dc13-2704.
20. Li TT, et al. Prevalence and clinical characteristics of non-alcoholic fatty liver disease in newly diagnosed patients with ketosis-onset diabetes. Diabetes Metab. 2018. https://doi.org/10.1016/j.diabet.2018.03.002.
21. Harman DJ, et al. Prevalence and natural history of histologically proven chronic liver disease in a longitudinal cohort of patients with type 1 diabetes. Hepatology. 2014;60:158–68. https://doi.org/10.1002/hep.27098.
22. Cusi K, et al. Non-alcoholic fatty liver disease (NAFLD) prevalence and its metabolic associations in patients with type 1 diabetes and type 2 diabetes. Diabetes Obes Metab. 2017;19:1630–4. https://doi.org/10.1111/dom.12973.
23. Llaurado G, et al. Liver fat content and hepatic insulin sensitivity in overweight patients with type 1 diabetes. J Clin Endocrinol Metab. 2015;100:607–16. https://doi.org/10.1210/jc.2014-3050.
24. Petit JM, et al. Type 1 diabetes is not associated with an increased prevalence of hepatic steatosis. Diabet Med. 2015;32:1648–51. https://doi.org/10.1111/dme.12805.
25. Schwimmer JB, et al. Effect of a low free sugar diet vs usual diet on nonalcoholic fatty liver disease in adolescent boys: a randomized clinical trial. JAMA. 2019;321:256–65. https://doi.org/10.1001/jama.2018.20579.
26. Van Name MA, et al. A low omega-6 to omega-3 PUFA ratio (n-6:n-3 PUFA) diet to treat fatty liver disease in obese youth. J Nutr. 2020. https://doi.org/10.1093/jn/nxaa183.
27. Lavine JE, et al. Effect of vitamin E or metformin for treatment of nonalcoholic fatty liver disease in children and adolescents: the TONIC randomized controlled trial. JAMA. 2011;305:1659–68. https://doi.org/10.1001/jama.2011.520.
28. Schwimmer JB, et al. In children with nonalcoholic fatty liver disease, cysteamine bitartrate delayed release improves liver enzymes but does not reduce disease activity scores. Gastroenterology. 2016;151:1141–1154.e1149. https://doi.org/10.1053/j.gastro.2016.08.027.
29. Belfort R, et al. A placebo-controlled trial of pioglitazone in subjects with nonalcoholic steatohepatitis. N Engl J Med. 2006;355:2297–307. https://doi.org/10.1056/NEJMoa060326.
30. Armstrong MJ, et al. Liraglutide safety and efficacy in patients with nonalcoholic steatohepatitis (LEAN): a multicentre, double-blind, randomised, placebo-controlled phase 2 study. Lancet. 2016;387:679–90. https://doi.org/10.1016/s0140-6736(15)00803-x.
31. Dong Y, et al. Efficacy and safety of glucagon-like peptide-1 receptor agonists in non-alcoholic fatty liver disease: a systematic review and meta-analysis. Clin Res Hepatol Gastroenterol. 2017;41:284–95. https://doi.org/10.1016/j.clinre.2016.11.009.
32. Eriksson JW, et al. Effects of dapagliflozin and n-3 carboxylic acids on non-alcoholic fatty liver disease in people with type 2 diabetes: a

double-blind randomised placebo-controlled study. Diabetologia. 2018;61:1923–34. https://doi.org/10.1007/s00125-018-4675-2.

33. Kuchay MS, et al. Effect of empagliflozin on liver fat in patients with type 2 diabetes and nonalcoholic fatty liver disease: a randomized controlled trial (E-LIFT trial). Diabetes Care. 2018;41:1801–8. https://doi.org/10.2337/dc18-0165.

18 Current Treatment of Pediatric Type 2 Diabetes

Stephanie Samuels, Michelle Van Name, Cindy Guandalini, William V. Tamborlane, and Sonia Caprio

Overview

Treatment of pediatric type 2 diabetes is relatively "new," being first described approximately 25 years ago [1]. In association with the epidemic of childhood obesity, today's youth are being diagnosed with T2D much more frequently. Pediatric T2D is uncommonly diagnosed prior to 10 years of age and is more commonly observed in adolescent girls than boys (usually in a 2:1 ratio). Screening of overweight and obese youngsters by oral glucose tolerance testing with or without measurement of a HbA1c level

S. Samuels (✉) · M. Van Name · C. Guandalini · W. V. Tamborlane
S. Caprio
Yale-New Haven Children's Hospital, Department of Pediatrics, Yale School of Medicine, New Haven, CT, USA
e-mail: stephanie.samuels@yale.edu

W. V. Tamborlane (ed.), *Diabetes in Children and Adolescents*, Contemporary Endocrinology,
https://doi.org/10.1007/978-3-030-64133-7_18

have identified youngsters who can be managed initially with an intensive diet and exercise intervention alone. Conversely, other youth diagnosed with T2D present with either DKA or hyperglycemic hyperosmolar syndrome and require initial treatment with insulin.

Despite large variations in symptoms at the time of diagnosis of T2D in adolescents, the disorder consists of two major factors: severe insulin resistance due to obesity and emerging pubertal development in combination with progressive β-cell failure in the absence of antibodies directed at components of β-cells. Age between 10 years and older, obesity, and negative anti-β-cell antibodies are the hallmarks that differentiate T2D from T1D. In the United States, T2D is being increasingly recognized in children in certain ethnic groups such as Native Americans, African Americans, and Latino Americans who represent more than half of newly diagnosed cases in some US medical centers. These patients often have a family history of type 2 diabetes, acanthosis nigricans, and poor metabolic control that predisposes them to the earlier appearance of microvascular and macrovascular complications.

Treatment of Pediatric T2D

As noted previously, many youth diagnosed with T2D require initial treatment with insulin to rapidly reverse gluco-toxicity. This also provides clinicians with the opportunity to initiate insulin treatment while awaiting results of pancreatic antibody test results to determine whether the obese youngster has T1D or T2D. Fortunately, almost all of the T2D patients can be weaned off insulin and switched to twice-a-day dosing with metformin.

Metformin is a biguanide medication that was approved for use in youth with T2D in 1999, making it a well-established treatment for pediatric T2D [2]. Metformin decreases hepatic glucose production, improves hepatic insulin sensitivity, impacts gut microbiome, raises GLP-1 levels, and limits inflammation. When initiating treatment with metformin, renal function should first be assessed as metformin is cleared by the kidneys, and toxic increases in circulating metformin levels have been reported to be related to the development of lactic acidosis in patients with reduced glomerular filtration rates. For the same reason, it is recommended that metformin should be held in case there is a decline in renal function due to administration of intravenous contrast materials, as well as during periods of dehydration.

When initiating metformin therapy, the dose of metformin is slowly titrated upwards to mitigate against unpleasant gastrointestinal side effects. It can be initiated with a single daily dose of 500 mg at either breakfast or dinner. A second dose is added with the other meal after 1 week, though slower titration may be required if gastrointestinal side effects have not yet resolved. Each week an additional dose is added, or more slowly if needed, until patients are taking 1000 mg with breakfast and 1000 mg with dinner. However, not all patients are able to titrate up to these maximally tolerated doses. An immediate release formulation is available in 500, 850, and 1000 mg tablets, and there is also as a 500 mg/5 mL oral solution. An extended release formulation is also available, in tablets of 500, 750, and 1000 mg. The extended release formulation is favored by some patients due to fewer gastrointestinal side effects when compared to the immediate release tablets. The extended release formulation should also be considered as an alternate treatment strategy, particularly for youth who do not routinely eat breakfast or who have difficulty taking medications twice a day. Given that metformin is a cornerstone of T2D therapy and T2D is strongly inherited, parents and children with T2D who are both taking metformin can take their doses in tandem to provide support and supervision for each other.

Abdominal discomfort, nausea, and diarrhea are the most common adverse effects of metformin, especially early in treatment. As discussed previously, these issues can be mitigated by dosing metformin with meals and slowly titrating metformin to maximally tolerated doses. It is noteworthy that these complaints wane over time with stable or temporarily reduced dosing. Metformin use for long-term treatment has also been associated with B12 deficiency in adults, leading some clinicians to monitor B12 levels annually and/or recommend prophylactic treatment with a multivitamin. One beneficial potential side effect of metformin is weight loss, which has been reported in adolescents with overweight/obesity. A recent study examined the efficacy and safety of metformin as an adjunctive treatment with insulin in overweight adolescents with T1D. While metformin treatment was well tolerated and was associated with modest weight loss, no improvement in metabolic control was observed [3].

The TODAY study demonstrated that most youth with T2D who have been weaned off insulin can be well controlled with metformin alone early in the course of the disease [4]. However, after starting with a mean A1c of 5.9% at baseline, almost 50% of TODAY study participants treated with metformin alone increased A1C levels to >8.0% within approximately 12 months. Consequently, the rapid failure of metformin monotherapy required rescue treatment with insulin, the only other drug that had been approved by the FDA for use in youth with T2D [5]. The inconvenient truth is that most youth with T2D do not do well with insulin treatment alone or in combination with metformin.

Insulin

Add-on therapy with insulin is often required with increasing duration of diabetes. In contrast to youth with T1D, youth with T2D may require only basal insulin to improve glycemic control, as rescue treatment if metformin monotherapy fails. Initial dosing of basal insulin is 0.25–0.5 units/kg/day and then titrated up as necessary. The long-acting insulin analogs (glargine and detemir) have replaced NPH insulin for basal insulin treatment and degludec, the first ultra-long-acting insulin analog, is being increasingly used. Indeed, we recently reported that switching poorly controlled youth with T2D to degludec was an effective means to lower HbA1c levels [6]. In contrast, youth with T1D in our diabetes clinics showed no improvement in metabolic control when switched to insulin degludec (Table 18.1).

Since virtually all youth with T2D are overweight or markedly obese, concentrated insulins are also a helpful tool to address the high doses of insulin that may be required in these patients. In addition to the 100 unit/ml preparations, glargine pens are avail-

Table 18.1 Lowering HbA1c with insulin degludec in T2D but not T1D

HbA1c (%)	0 months	3 months	6 months
Type 2 diabetes ($n = 82$)	10.1%	10.0%	10.1%
Type 1 diabetes ($n = 16$)	10.6%	9.7%	8.3%

From Elahi et al. [6], with permission

able in a 300 unit/ml concentration and degludec pens are available in a 200 unit/ml concentration. Larger insulin doses that can be administered in a single injection may be a more realistic way to optimize compliance in adolescents than administration of twice-a-day doses of basal insulin. U300 glargine also has a longer duration of action compared to equivalent doses of U100 glargine.

The American Diabetes Association (ADA) and the International Society for Pediatric and Adolescent Diabetes (ISPAD) have recommend that a goal of treatment of youth with T2D and T1D should be to achieve and maintain HbA1c levels <7.5%. Many pediatric patients with T2D can reach a target of <6.5% after initial treatment is optimized. However, if this target is not reached with basal insulin with or without metformin in youth with T2D, clinicians should add boluses of rapid-acting insulin to the regimen. Bolus insulins include rapid-acting insulin aspart, lispro, and glulisine. Insulin lispro is available in a concentrated 200 unit/ml form and Fiasp is a faster-acting insulin aspart. Dosing of rapid-acting insulins is variable and should be individualized to the patient's needs. One approach to pre-meal bolus dosing is to start with the largest meal of the day, with coverage for other meals added as needed. Importantly, in youth with T2D who maintain some β-cell function, finely titrated pre-meal bolus dosing may not be necessary due to the impact of residual endogenous insulin production on managing postprandial hyperglycemia. Simplified dosing, for example fixed 30-unit doses with each meal, may be preferable and a more realistic management plan for some youth.

Pre-mixed insulins (fixed ratios of rapid-acting and intermediate-acting insulins) given once or twice a day are often used in adolescents with T2D. Here again, residual β-cell function can compensate for insulin to glucose mismatches that occur in the absence of bolus insulin. Pre-mixed insulins are a valuable tool for youth in whom basal bolus dosing is a challenge, and may be used strategically for patients who eat intermittently throughout the day.

The Pediatric Diabetes Consortium (PDC) recently compared differences between adolescents with T1D and T2D. In that study, youth with T2D were more likely to be female, overweight/obese, and from low-income, minority families; whereas, adolescents with T1D were more likely to present with diabetic ketoacidosis and have higher mean HbA_{1c} levels at diagnosis. More than 70% in both cohorts achieved target HbA_{1c} levels <7.5% within 6 months, but fewer participants with T1D than T2D could maintain target HbA_{1c} levels after 6 months consistently throughout 3 years post diagnosis. Moreover, of the 401 participants with T2D with ≥24 months diabetes duration on enrolment in the registry, 47% required no insulin treatment. Median C-peptide levels were 1.43 mmol/l in the subset of participants with T2D but only 0.06 mmol/l in the subset with T1D [7, 8]. Thus, although families of children and adolescents with T2D face greater socioeconomic obstacles and risk factors for poor diabetes outcomes, the greater retention of residual endogenous insulin secretion likely contributes to the increased ability of children and adolescents with type 2 diabetes to maintain target HbA_{1c} during the first 3 years of diabetes diagnosis.

It remains to be determined why HbA1c levels are markedly increased in many adolescents with T2D after 2–4 years of treatment, despite C-peptide levels that are elevated and in the face of treatment with both metformin and insulin. Continued weight gain and severe insulin resistance have been suggested as playing important roles. Moreover, non-compliance is a common contributing cause of failure of metformin treatment in teenagers with T2D. In these patients, add-on treatment with only basal insulin may be too difficult to manage. It is not coincidental that the PDC T2D Registry has shown that youth with T2D who require insulin rescue are rarely able to lower A1c levels to <7.5%. Thus, the large majority of pediatric T2D patients with longer duration of treatment are desperately in need of new treatment options that go beyond metformin and insulin.

Why Have So Many Clinical Trials of New Drugs for Youth with T2D Failed?

Prior to 2019, metformin was the only agent the US Food and Drug Administration approved for use in the treatment of youth with type 2 diabetes based on the results of a pivotal (although small) phase 3 clinical trial that was completed in 1999. Insulin is also approved for use in pediatric type 2 diabetes. However, this approval was not the result of a pediatric study but by extrapolation from the efficacy of insulin in adults with T2D and youth with T1D. Despite the plethora of new drugs in several new drug classes, only one new drug has been approved for use in pediatric diabetes and that was only in the past year [9]. The reluctance of regulatory agencies to extrapolate the efficacy of new drugs approved for adults with T2D to include adolescents is one reason why only metformin and insulin were approved for use in youth with T2D for more than 20 years.

There were many reasons why pivotal phase 3 trials have been failing to enroll, randomize, and retain enough participants to determine the efficacy and safety of new drugs for treatment of youth with type 2 diabetes. An early obstacle was that regulatory agencies required initial pharmacokinetic and pharmacodynamic dose-finding studies to ensure that subsequent phase 3 trial testing doses approved for use in adults did not expose youngsters to toxic levels of these new drugs. There were two main reasons why this requirement was problematic. First, even straightforward, single-dose pharmacokinetic and pharmacodynamic studies that required a relatively small number of subjects took 2–4 years to complete. Even worse, such studies were unnecessary because pediatric T2D is restricted to older children and adolescents aged 10 to <18 years who are overweight or obese. Consequently, drug exposures in all these pediatric pharmacokinetic and pharmacodynamic studies were similar to or lower than drug exposures in adults because the body weight of pediatric participants was the same or greater than adults with T2D. Based on this experience, preliminary pharmacokinetic and pharmacodynamic studies are no longer required.

A current problem is that there are simply too many studies required by the regulatory agencies in a population of patients that is still relatively small. Due to the epidemic of childhood obesity in the United States, America has one of the largest populations of youth with T2D. However, more than 90% of patients in the United States come from disadvantaged, low socioeconomic families and parents cannot afford to miss work to attend frequent study visits. Potential subjects for these clinical trials often miss-scheduled clinic visits or are lost to follow-up, and many struggle with adherence to taking medications and carrying out other diabetes-related tasks. In addition, many patients are excluded from these studies due to behavioral problems, depression, other psychiatric disorders, and use of atypical antipsychotic medications. Moreover, minority parents are often leery of research.

Eligibility criteria mandated by regulatory authorities have compounded these challenges and made successful recruitment of subjects virtually impossible by excluding 50–90% of potential participants. In addition, protocols developed by sponsors and endorsed by regulatory agencies have included unnecessary barriers for participation, such as frequent visits to measure morning fasting glucose levels. Finally, clinical trial budgets offered by CROs/sponsors to the Clinical Centers are often inadequate to cover the costs of carrying out the protocols, as well as the many activities required to launch and close out the study. Indeed, there are many other reasons why academic investigators in the United States were not interested in participating in these studies, especially working alone, as a single center with limited institutional support [10].

A New Consortium Approach to Completing Clinical Trials for Pediatric T2D

An aim of the Pediatric Diabetes Consortium (PDC) is to utilize the resources of the PDC Coordinating Center and Executive Committee to improve study protocols, centralize interactions with sponsors, and oversee the performance of PDC Clinical

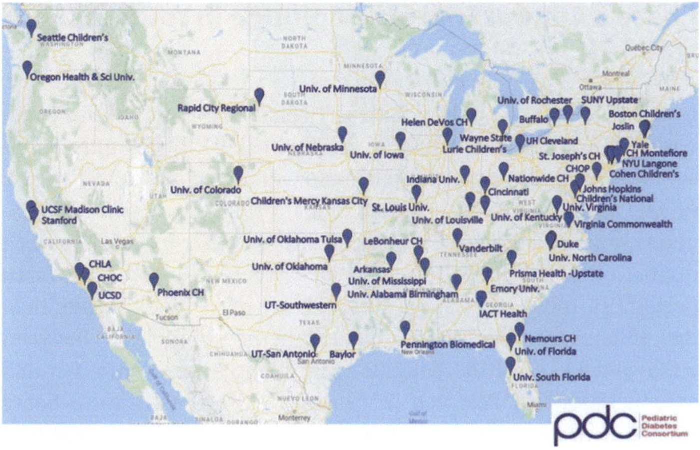

Fig. 18.1 Map of PDC Clinical Centers on 1/1/2020

Centers, all of whom have committed themselves to work together as a group rather than individual centers (Fig. 18.1). Key features include a Consulting Group to improve protocol design; Master Service Agreements between the Coordinating Center and Clinical Centers covering confidentiality agreements and contract language; negotiation of a standard Site Budget with Contract Research Organizations (CROs)/Sponsors that reflect actual Clinical Center costs; Weekly Conference Calls with CROs/Sponsors to track progress of Clinical Center launches; and Monthly Oversight Calls with investigators and study Coordinators to track Clinical Center performance, discuss enrollment strategies, and identify emerging problems.

The Consortium model played a key role in the completion of the pivotal trial of liraglutide for treatment of youth with T2D, and PDC centers have played a pivotal role in exceeding the projected number of randomized subjects needed by two pediatric T2D studies that are nearing completion. While the Consortium model is still a work in progress, PDC has more recently assisted in the successful launch of new T2D studies, and negotiations are in underway for PDC participation in other diabetes-related studies.

Phase 3 Clinical Trial of Liraglutide in Youth with T2D

Liraglutide is the first drug that has been approved for use in youth with T2D, since metformin in 1999. In the Ellipse study sponsored by Novo Nordisk, patients who were 10 to less than 17 years of age were randomly assigned, in a 1:1 ratio, to receive subcutaneous liraglutide (up to 1.8 mg per day) or placebo for a 26-week double-blind period, followed by a 26-week open-label extension period [9]. Inclusion criteria were a body mass index greater than the 85th percentile and a glycated hemoglobin level between 7.0% and 11.0% if the patients were being treated with diet and exercise alone or between 6.5% and 11.0% if they were being treated with metformin (with or without insulin). All the patients received metformin during the trial. The primary endpoint was the change from baseline in the glycated hemoglobin level after 26 weeks. Secondary end points included the change in fasting plasma glucose level. Safety was assessed throughout the course of the trial.

After more than 4 years of recruitment, a total of 135 patients underwent randomization; 134 received at least one dose of liraglutide (66 patients) or placebo (68 patients). Demographic characteristics were similar in the two groups. At the 26-week analysis of the primary efficacy end point, the mean glycated hemoglobin level had decreased by 0.64 percentage points with liraglutide and increased by 0.42 percentage points with placebo. For an estimated treatment difference of −1.06 percentage points ($P < 0.001$), the difference increased to −1.30 percentage points by 52 weeks (Fig. 18.2). Fasting plasma glucose level had decreased at both time points in the liraglutide group but had increased in the placebo group. The number of patients who reported adverse events was similar in the two groups (56 [84.8%] with liraglutide and 55 [80.9%] with placebo), but the overall rates of adverse events and gastrointestinal adverse events were higher with liraglutide. Thus, in children and adolescents with T2D, liraglutide, at a dose of up to 1.8 mg per day was efficacious in improving glycemic control over 52 weeks.

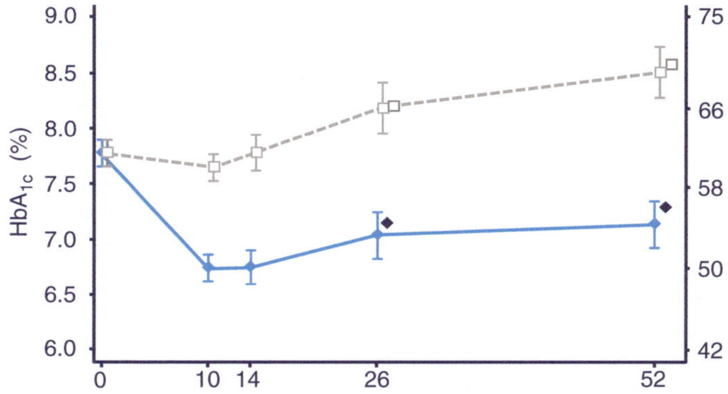

Fig. 18.2 Change from baseline in the liraglutide group (blue) versus placebo (gray). (From Tamborlane et al. [9], with permission)

The results of this study led to the approval of use of liraglutide by the US Food and Drug Administration in 2019, which has been followed by the near completion of several other clinical trials of new drugs for the treatment of pediatric T2D. We anticipate that these new drug approvals will transform the treatment of T2D in children and adolescents.

References

1. Pinhas-Hamiel O, Dolan LM, Daniels SR, Standiford D, Khoury PR, Zeitler P. Increased incidence of non-insulin-dependent diabetes mellitus among adolescents. J Pediatr. 1996;128:608–15.
2. Jones KL, Arslanian S, Peterokova VA, Park JS, Tomlinson MJ. Effect of metformin in pediatric patients with type 2 diabetes: a randomized controlled trial. Diabetes Care. 2002;25:89–94.
3. Libman IM, Miller KM, DiMeglio LA, et al. Effect of metformin added to insulin on glycemic control among overweight/obese adolescents with type 1 diabetes: a randomized clinical trial. JAMA. 2015;314:2241–50.
4. TODAY Study Group. Metformin monotherapy in youth with recent onset type 2 diabetes: experience from the pre-randomization run-in phase of the TODAY study. Pediatr Diabetes. 2012;13:369–73.
5. TODAY Study Group. A clinical trial to maintain glycemic control in youth with type 2 diabetes. N Engl J Med. 2012;366:2247–56.

6. Elahi S, Patel AD, Guandalini C, Steffen A, Sherr J, Tamborlane WV, Van Name MA. Impact of switching youth with diabetes to insulin degludec in clinical practice. Endocr Pract. 2019;25:226–9.
7. Gregg B, Connor CG, Cheng P, et al. C-peptide levels in pediatric type 2 diabetes in the Pediatric Diabetes Consortium T2D Clinic Registry. Pediatr Diabetes. 2016;17:274–80.
8. Van Name MA, Cheng P, Gal RL, Kollman C, Lynch J, Nelson B, Tamborlane WV. Youth with type 1 and type 2 diabetes in the Pediatric Diabetes Consortium (PDC) Registries: comparing clinical characteristics and glycemic control diabetes. Medicine. 2020;37:863–7.
9. Tamborlane WV, Fainberg U, Frimer-Larsen H, Hafez M, Hale PM, Jalaludin MY, Kovarenko M, Libman I, Lynch J, Rao PV, Shehadeh N, Turan S, Weghuber D, Barrientos-Pérez M, Barrett T. Liraglutide in children and adolescents with type 2 diabetes. NEJM. 2019;381:637–46.
10. Farrell R, Bethin K, Klingensmith G, Tamborlane WV, Gubitosi-Klug R. Barriers to participation in industry-sponsored clinical trials in pediatric type 2 diabetes. Pediatr Diabetes. 2017;18:574–8.

19 The Yale Bright Bodies Lifestyle Intervention Program: An Intensive Lifestyle Intervention for Obese Children and Adolescents With and Without T2D

Mary Savoye, Paulina Rose, Stephanie Samuels, William V. Tamborlane, Sonia Caprio, and Michelle Van Name

M. Savoye (✉) · P. Rose · S. Samuels · W. V. Tamborlane · S. Caprio
M. Van Name
Yale-New Haven Children's Hospital, Department of Pediatrics, Yale School of Medicine, New Haven, CT, USA
e-mail: mayr.savoye@yale.edu

W. V. Tamborlane (ed.), *Diabetes in Children and Adolescents*, Contemporary Endocrinology,
https://doi.org/10.1007/978-3-030-64133-7_19

Background

The Yale Bright Bodies Lifestyle Intervention (BB LSI) was developed to fill the unmet needs of obese, inner city children with or without T2D from disadvantaged families. This family-based, lifestyle intervention has been an ongoing treatment option for families in New Haven CT for more than 20 years. The program has several complimentary elements that contribute to the success of our youngsters. Subjects are referred to our program by clinicians from our Pediatric Obesity Clinics, the Yale Primary Care Center, and from pediatricians in the Greater New Haven area: obese youth with or without T2D are eligible to participate in the program.

Setting of Bright Bodies Lifestyle Intervention (BB LSI)

Participants 7–16 years old and at least one parent/caregiver in the BB LSI attend the program at a local public school twice a week for one or more 12-week sessions. All sessions are held in the evening after school and after the parents' work. The local school setting was chosen due to limitations in transportation options of our socioeconomically diverse families. We also anticipated that suburban families outside of New Haven would not want to travel long distances two times per week to participate in the program, although many have chosen to do so. A second, inner city setting was later developed to better serve our Spanish-speaking population who lived in a predominantly Hispanic neighborhood in New Haven.

Program Format

The program consists of supervised exercise of 50 minutes twice a week and nutrition/behavior modification (30 minutes/session for 7–10 year olds; 40 minutes for 11–16 year olds) once a week. Participants and caregivers attend all nutrition-related topics together; whereas, behavior modification classes for participants and caregivers are held separately. Participants are weighed approximately every 1–2 weeks, and weight checks are mandatory at the beginning and end of the 12-week program. Caregivers are also encouraged to be weighed to show support for their child. During the first randomized controlled trial (RCT) of our lifestyle intervention [1], the program met twice a week for the first 6 months and then every other week for the last 6 months to model the active and maintenance phases, respectively.

Program Components

Behavior Modification Component of the BB LSI

The behavior modification component of the program is facilitated by our registered dietitian and social worker. Topics are provided from the Smart Moves curriculum, which was developed by Mary Savoye, one of the authors of this chapter. Behavior modification topics included *Ready, Set, Goal; Risky Business: Identifying High Risk Situations*; *Environmental Engineering*; *Mirror, Mirror on the Wall; Bullies, Teasers, and Other Annoying People; Stress Management for the Stress Eater,* and *Oops I Slipped—Understanding a Relapse*. Methods include techniques such as self-awareness, goal setting, stimulus control, reframing, coping skills training (CST), and contingency management. The topic of Risky Business uses self-awareness to help a child identify an eating trigger, and CST allows the child to address the risk by perhaps roleplaying a risky situation with healthier, adaptive behavior in front of peers and receiving feedback.

Although parents or other caregivers attend the nutrition-topic classes with their child, they do not attend the behavior modification classes together, since this gives the child autonomy and allows for frank discussion to take place, which is ultimately more effective. Parents and caregivers attend their behavior modification classes separately in which the adults also appreciate. Behavior modification classes for caregivers include topics that reflect challenges parents verbalize. CST and brief solution-focused therapy (SOFT) are the primary techniques utilized. A pilot study using CST with overweight parents of children in our program showed positive outcome trends for parents when compared to those without CST. SOFT has also been shown to be an effective counseling strategy for family-based obesity interventions [2]. Its premise is to focus on what is working rather than what is not and to use innate qualities to help overcome challenges. Two fundamental activities of the group involve the use of strength cards (showing positive characteristics) to emphasize the unique attributes of their overweight child (Fig. 19.1) and writing letters about how life has improved. SOFT has been shown to empower caregivers of obese children [2] and it is one of the components of the BB LSI that emphasizes the importance of the parents' role in support and modeling healthy behaviors.

As a dynamic program, we update additional components every few years. Currently we are conducting a randomized clinical trial to determine if the addition of mindfulness for adolescents results in a greater decrease in BMI than the control group (i.e., traditional BB LSI). Briefly, mindfulness involves focusing of one's awareness on the present moment in a non-judgmental, accepting way. Children attend six weekly 40-minute sessions (caregivers are also welcome) in a quiet area away from the gymnasium delivered by a certified mindfulness instructor. In addition to BMI, we are also measuring perceived stress (via a questionnaire), physical stress (via salivary cortisol measurements), and food intake (calories, fat, sugar) before and after 6 weeks of mindfulness instruction. This addition to the program is being investigated due to the relationship between chronic stress and obesity and because many of our children and parents report high levels of stress, which may adversely impact their ability to make healthy lifestyle choices. If the addition of mindfulness shows greater improvement in BMI in adolescents, it will be added to the behavior modification component of the program.

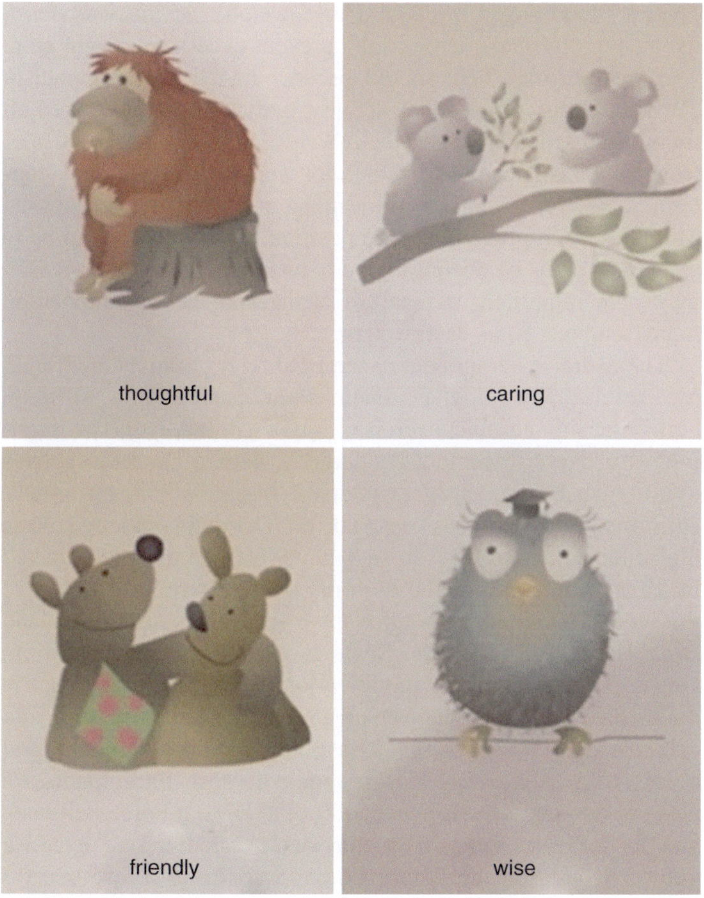

Fig. 19.1 Samples of strength cards used in parent classes

Exercise Component of the BB LSI

The importance of physical activity for overweight children with and without T2D cannot be overstated. Physical activity generally decreases blood glucose and burns calories, creating a win-win situation for the overweight/obese child with T2D who needs to control blood sugar levels and lose weight. At the very least, increasing physical exercise may prevent excessive weight gain. Thus, youth with T2D should be encouraged to participate in 30–60 minutes of physical activity daily and include strength training on at least 3 days/week. Weight training includes use of resistance bands or push-ups but not weightlifting which is contraindicated for youngsters. Indeed, an aim of increased physical activity is to improve body composition by increasing lean body mass, as well as by decreasing body fat mass [3]. This is a reason why it is important to measure changes in body composition rather than just changes in weight.

The exercise component of the BB LSI program is facilitated by exercise physiologists. Each class consists of a warmup, high-intensity aerobic exercise, and a cool down. The high-intensity exercise includes a large variety of games such as Swim Fish Swim, obstacle courses, basketball, flag football, sprinting games, and basic sport drills. The main objective of the high-intensity exercise is to sustain 65–80% of the age-adjusted maximal heart rate for the duration of the exercise. To achieve this goal, a heart rate monitor is worn by all participants and Borg's Perceived Exertion Scale is used to monitor exertion. However, instruction for modification accompanies each activity so that each child can keep up and increase their strength and exercise capacity gradually. The group is non-judgmental and every child is encouraged to try their hardest. Participants are also encouraged to exercise 3 additional days at home per week and to decrease sedentary behaviors. A challenging exercise video is found on the Bright Bodies website as a resource for additional activity; this video also offers instruction for modification.

Motivational tools are used to encourage regular attendance. For example, children accumulate points for each exercise class or activity throughout the program or may earn a "Bright Bodies Buck" (raffle ticket). To provide variety and enthusiasm, there are special exercise events such as dance offs, family yoga, and holiday-related activities such as turkey trots and monster mashes. The kids love these events.

Nutrition Education Component of the BB LSI

The nutrition education component of the program used a non-diet, Good Food Choices approach that emphasizes low-fat, nutrient-dense foods of moderate portion sizes. An initial sub-study analysis of the BB LSI comparing BMI z-scores in those using the non-diet approach versus a structured meal plan (i.e., a strict diet approach) showed favorable results at 1 year. Namely, during year one, "dieters" lost more weight than those using the non-diet approach but, by year 2, those utilizing the non-dieting approach continued to decrease BMI z-scores, while dieters rebounded towards baseline [4] (Fig. 19.2). The program's non-diet, Good Food Choices approach is the foundation of all nutrition topics, including *What's in Your Beverage?; Determining Portion Sizes, Better Food Choices: A Non-Diet Approach, Making Sense of a Food Labels, Bag It—The Pros to Bringing Lunch to School* and *Recipes Dear to Our Heart: Ingredient Substitutions for Traditional Recipes.* The initial nutrition class focuses on decreasing sugar-laden beverages for the entire family as this one change seems to have a significant impact on caloric intake and is a realistic first step for families.

Our registered dietitians use the *Smart Moves Workbook,* which provides a consistent structure for all topics. The first 12 weeks of the Program offers more nutrition topics, but by the

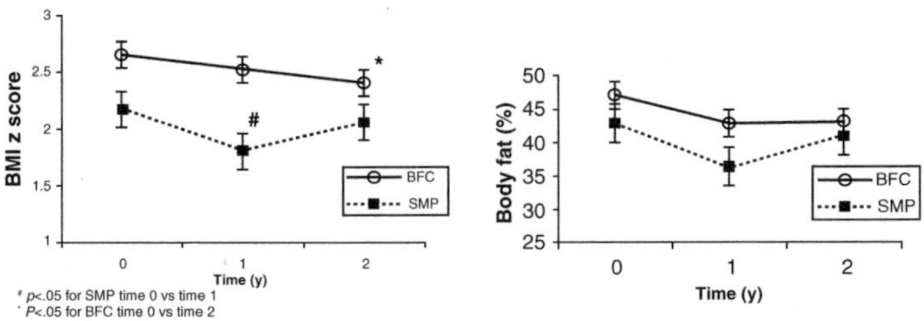

Fig. 19.2 BMI-z and % body fat change in diet versus non-diet approach. (From Savoye et al. [4], with permission)

Week 1	Orientation
Week 2	Group Dynamics and Goal Setting
Week 3	What's in Your Dink?
Week 4	Determining Portion Control
Week 5	Keeping Food Records
Week 6	Risky Business: Identifying Eating Triggers
Week 7	Risky Business: Coping with Eating Triggers
Week 8	Non-Diet Approach to Weight Management
Week 9	Label-Sense... Making Sense of a Food Label
Week 10	Bullies, Teasers, and Other Annoying People
Week 11	Bag It!
Week 12	Life in the Fast Lane

Fig. 19.3 First 12-week topics of Bright Bodies Program

second 12 weeks, there are equal behavior modification topics (Fig. 19.3). Additional information regarding good food choices are described for youth with T1D in Chap. 10.

Caregiver's Role in the BB LSI

When initiating a lifestyle intervention for the child or adolescent with or without T2DM, it is fundamental to include the parent or caregiver who is the agent of change in the home. The parent or caregiver generally purchases the food, prepares the food, and acts as a role model for the family unit. A family approach that offers support is crucial so the child does not feel singled out by other family members. The success of the child is therefore contingent upon the parent or caregiver's informed and active role of making lifestyle changes for the family. It is one of the main reasons why a parent or caregiver plays a key role in our BB LSI program.

Program Incentives

Bright Bodies Bucks

Because the initial goal of the program is to halt weight gain in these overweight children, we reinforce this by providing a "Bright Bodies Buck" for those who either stay the same or lose weight when they are weighed. A buck is basically a raffle ticket that goes into a bucket and gives them an opportunity to win a $20 gift card, every 3 weeks. Weight maintenance earns one buck, while weight loss earns two. Also, as stated earlier, the exercise component plays games in which children earn points and these points also result in receiving Bright Bodies Bucks. Another way to earn a Bright Bodies Buck is for a child to write an article in our newsletter, which is distributed towards the end of each 12-week cycle. The child is given the opportunity to write one or two paragraphs about how the Program has helped them or what they like best about the Program. The newsletter also includes a seasonal recipe, exercise tip, and a program update.

Certificates

We learned early on that most children (and adults!) want recognition for their hard work. A simple certificate with the child's name on it is given at the end of the 12 weeks in a ceremonial fashion. Each child comes up to receive the certificate and the families and staff members applaud them.

The Successes of the BB LSI Program

Anthropometrics and Metabolic Improvement

We have carried out several randomized clinical trials that have demonstrated the successes of the Yale BB LSI in overweight/obese youth with and without prediabetes or T2D. In a large, randomized trial published in JAMA in 2007 [1], we showed that the BB LSI had beneficial effects on body composition and increased insulin sensitivity in overweight children at 12 months. In contrast, the participants randomized to the clinic control group showed increases in weight, BMI, and body fat mass throughout the study. This study was followed up at 24 months, and the treatment effect was sustained [5].

We subsequently showed that compared with standard clinical care, the Yale Bright Bodies LSI was a more effective means of reducing the risk of T2D in obese adolescents with elevated 2-hour plasma glucose levels [5, 6]. Moreover, insulin sensitivity indices were significantly improved in Bright Body participants. More recently, we established that our BB LSI could also be adapted in adult women with obesity and prediabetes [7] (Fig. 19.4). In fact, the curriculum is currently being utilized for a study investigating BMI and cardiovascular outcomes in women with preeclampsia and eclampsia from delivery to 6 months post-

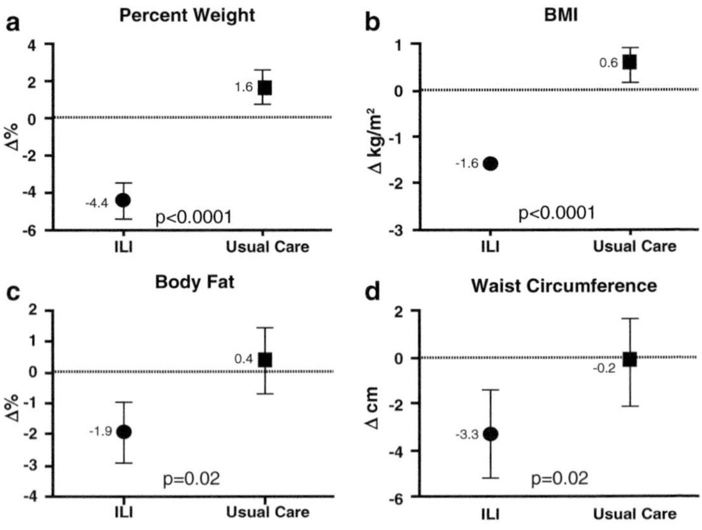

Fig. 19.4 Results of the Bright Bodies Intensive Lifestyle Intervention (ILI) versus Usual Care in a predominantly Hispanic population of obese women. (From Van Name et al. [7], with permission)

partum. Most recently, the program is being offered to adolescents on antipsychotics at a psychiatric hospital to mitigate weight gain as antipsychotics often result in significant obesity.

The BB LSI is also being utilized internationally, such as in Concepcion and Santiago Chile, and outcomes mirror those found in our early studies. Moreover, the Smart Moves curriculum is used throughout the United States in over 30 sites including universities, schools, reservations, government centers, and health clinics. A diabetes center in Kuwait has also started to utilize the Smart Moves Curriculum for obese children and adolescents with and without T2D.

Psychosocial Improvements

In addition to anthropometric and metabolic improvements, the Program has shown improved psychosocial measures. The Piers-Harris Self-Concept Scale (PHSCS) is a simple yes or no instrument with 80 questions that is filled out by the child. It measures how the child sees themselves and includes six categories: Behavioral Adjustment; Intellectual and School Status; Physical Appearance and Attributes; Freedom from Anxiety; Popularity; and Happiness and Satisfaction. Higher total scores indicate higher self-esteem. Total scores before and after the program showed statistically significant increases after 6 months of the BB LSI [4].

Because ours is a family-based program with a fair amount of time spent on the importance of good communication and support, we also measure family functioning using the McMaster Family Assessment Device (FAD). This questionnaire is completed by the parents who rate how well each statement describes their family (strongly agree to strongly disagree). Subscales for this questionnaire include Problem Solving, Communication, Roles (division of responsibility), Affective Responses (expression of love and other feelings), Affective Involvement (interest in one another), Behavior Control (how behavioral standards were expressed and maintained), and General Functioning (family functioning overall). In 2016, we determined that baseline self-esteem and family functioning moderated treatment effects. Specifically, BB LSI outperformed regular clinical care in youth with low self-esteem and poorly functioning families; whereas, youth with high self-esteem and high family functioning did well in either group [8]. These findings indicate that BB LSI is particularly beneficial for youth with low self-esteem and poorly functioning families.

Modest Weight Losses for Improved Blood Glucose Control

Although weight management is only one part of the treatment of the obese child, those with prediabetes and T2D can improve blood glucose levels significantly with even modest weight loss. Countless children and adolescents enrolled in the Yale BB LSI have lost weight, and those with T2D have improved their glucose control. Yale BB LSI success stories include modest weight loses to stories in which adolescents have lost over 100 pounds. Interestingly, in both of these extreme scenarios, we have had adolescents with T2D who were able to discontinue their metformin and rapid-acting insulin regimens.

An Illustrative Examples

An 11-year-old Nicole was initially treated for T2D with metformin monotherapy, but rapid-acting insulin was added due to metformin monotherapy failure. Her family was too overwhelmed to provide the insulin injections for Nicole, so the VNA visited her house twice per day to administer the injections. Subsequently, her participation in the BB LSI resulted in weight loss of 16 pounds and she was able to discontinue both medications. Even more impressive was 13-year-old Eric who lost over 120 pounds and came off both medications after an initial 40-pound loss. He stayed with the program until he was

18 years old, then went off to college and he has been able to maintain normal weight. Eric returns every year to talk with the children. In fact, many past patients volunteer to come back (some are now in their 30's) and share their success stories with newer members, which is a sentiment of belonging, gratitude, and long-term weight loss.

Personal Comments from Our Children and Families

After each 12-week session, parents and participants provide us with feedback about the program or how the program has changed their child. Some of these comments include the following.

Parents:

- My son finally has friends!
- This is the only place I see my child smile!
- He is so excited to come here that he gets ready an hour before we have to leave.
- Have you thought about offering the program on Saturdays?
- Have you thought about having the program every night instead of just two nights/week?
- My daughter is finally talking to me!

Kids:

- I run like a cheetah now! (8 years old)I am not failing gym class anymore! (14 years old)
- I don't spend as much time on video games. (15 years old)
- I made a lot of friends here. (12 years old)
- My family is nicer to me. (13 years old)
- I cook with my family now. (10 years old)
- I wear cooler clothes now. (16 years old)
- I think I'm going to go to college now. (15 years old)
- I tried out for softball and made the team! (14 years old)

Summary

The BB LSI is an evidence-based lifestyle intervention developed at Yale to meet the needs of our ethnically diverse population. It has shown decreases in BMI, percent body fat, and glucose levels, as well as increases in self-esteem and family functioning. It is a dynamic program that continues to add components based upon the needs of our patients and research evidence. Families and children have shared positive feedback over the years confirming that the program is well accepted and effective.

References

1. Savoye M, Shaw M, Dziura J, Rose P, Guandalini C, Goldberg-Gell R, Burgert T, Cali A, Zern T, Tamborlane WV, Caprio S. Clinical benefits of the Yale Bright Bodies intensive lifestyle intervention program in overweight children: a randomized control trial. JAMA. 2007;297:2697–704.
2. Nowicka P, Savoye M, Fisher PA. Which psychological method is most effective for group treatment? Int J Pediatr Obes. 2011;6(1):70–3.
3. DeStefano R, Caprio S, Fahey J, Tamborlane WV. Beneficial effects of supervised physical training in the management of overweight boys. Pediatr Diabetes. 2000;1:61–5.
4. Savoye M, Berry D, Dziura J, Shaw M, Serrecchia JB, Barbetta G, Rose P, Lavietes S, Caprio S. Anthropometric and psychosocial changes in obese adolescents enrolled in a weight management program. J Am Diet Assoc. 2005;105:364–70.
5. Savoye M, Nowicka P, Shaw M, Yu S, Dziura J, Chavent G, O'Malley G, Serrechia J, Tamborlane WV, Caprio S. Long-term results of a randomized controlled trial of a weight management program in an ethnically-diverse population of obese children. Pediatrics. 2011;127:402–10.
6. Savoye M, Caprio S, Dziura J, Camp A, Germain G, Summers C, Li F, Shaw M, Kursawe R, DePourcq F, Kim G, Tamborlane WV. Reversal of early abnormalities in glucose metabolism in obese youth: results of an intensive lifestyle randomized controlled trial. Diabetes Care. 2014;37:317–24.
7. Van Name MA, Camp A, Magenheimer E, Li F, Dziura JD, Montosa M, Patel A, Tamborlane WV. Effective translation of an intensive lifestyle intervention in prediabetic Hispanic women in a community health center setting. Diabetes Care. 2016;39:525–31.
8. Taylor JH, Xu Y, Li F, Shaw M, Dzuria J, Caprio S, Tamborlane WV, Nowicka P, Savoye M. Self-esteem and family functioning as predictors and moderators of treatment outcomes in ethnically-diverse obese youth with abnormal glucose tolerance. Pediatr Obes. 2017;12:453–61.

The Yale Children's Diabetes Program

20

What You Need to Know When Newly Diagnosed

Kerry Stephenson

K. Stephenson (✉)
Yale-New Haven Children's Hospital, Department of Pediatrics,
Yale School of Medicine, New Haven, CT, USA
e-mail: kerry.stephenson@yale.edu

W. V. Tamborlane (ed.), *Diabetes in Children and Adolescents*, Contemporary Endocrinology,
https://doi.org/10.1007/978-3-030-64133-7_20

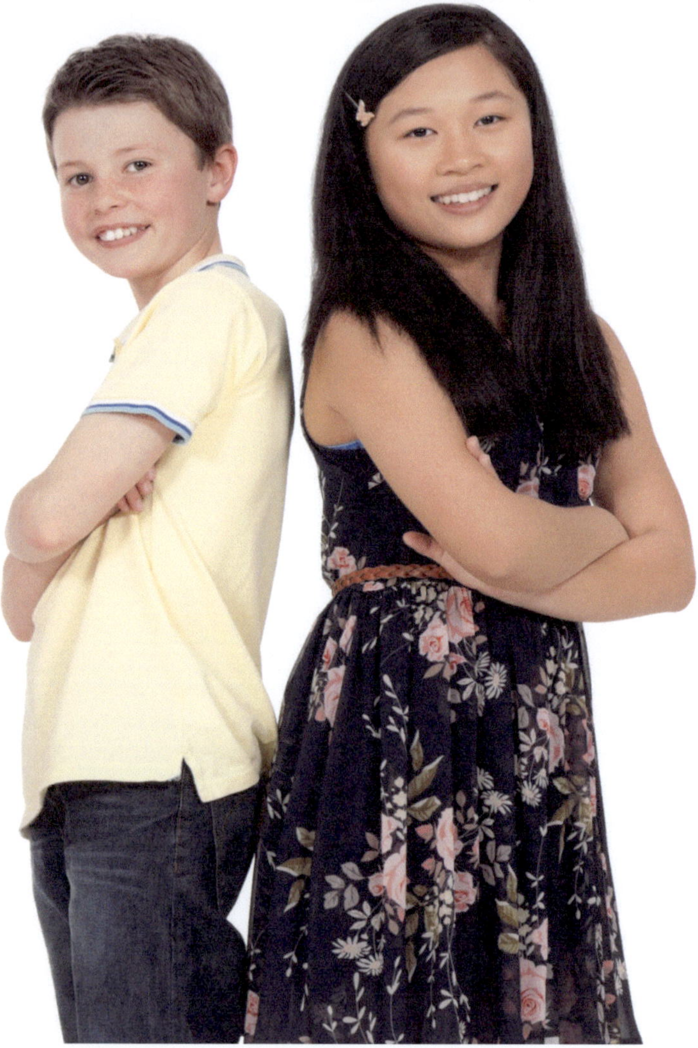

The Yale Children's Diabetes Program

Welcome

Need to Know

We know it can be hard to remember all the information you are learning. We have created these "Need to Know" sidebars at the beginning of each chapter to highlight the most important information.

In this book, we use the term "You" to mean:

- YOU, the child/teen with diabetes
- YOU, the brother/sister of the person with diabetes
- YOU, the parent/guardian of the person with diabetes
- YOU, the loved one of the person with diabetes

We want everyone who knows and loves the child/teen that is newly diagnosed to feel welcome to learn about diabetes. We hope that this book will foster this feeling. Please let us know if you need more than one copy, we are happy to provide extras.

If you are reading this book for the first time, you or someone you love has just been diagnosed with diabetes. We understand that this can be a very scary time and that there is a lot of information to learn before you go home. It may seem overwhelming and you might think you will never remember everything you are being taught.

The first thing we want you to do is TAKE A DEEP BREATH AND LET IT OUT SLOWLY.

You are not alone. Our team has worked with thousands of newly diagnosed families and we understand how difficult this time is. Please know that we are here to support you as you adjust to this "new normal." Believe it or not, you will create a "new normal" for your family. It will not happen overnight but, rest assured, there will be a time within the first year after the diagnosis that you will look back and be amazed at how far you have come.

In the meantime, here are a few of the ways that our team will help your family with this adjustment:

- You will have the chance to meet with our doctors, nurse practitioners, nutritionists, social workers, and nurses while in the hospital.
- This book is yours to keep, feel free to write notes or questions in it.
- A member of our team will speak to you every day when you leave the hospital, typically until your first follow-up visit.
- We will see you in our clinic about 2 weeks days after you leave the hospital and again 4–6 weeks later.
- We will see you in clinic every 3 months after that.
- We have team members available by phone for diabetes emergencies 24/7 and other team members are available via phone, email, and MyChart for non-urgent issues.

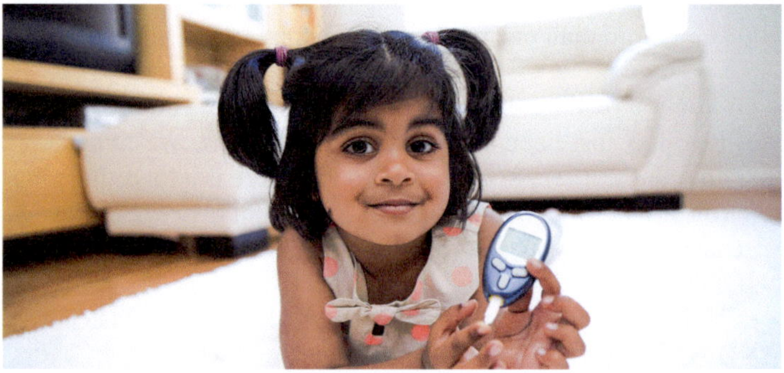

A Note from William Tamborlane, MD, Chief – Pediatric Endocrinology

I started my training in Pediatric Endocrinology in 1975 in an era that I like to classify as the "bad old days of type 1 diabetes." During that era, insulin was made from cow and pig pancreases and there was no good way to monitor blood sugar levels as blood glucose meters or hemoglobin A1c tests had not been developed.

Things began to change quickly in 1979–1981 when methods were developed to test blood sugar levels at home, track the hemoglobin A1c, and give insulin through a pump.

In 1993, the Diabetes Control and Complications Trial (DCCT) conclusively demonstrated that getting A1c levels as close to normal as possible significantly reduces the risk of complications from diabetes. In 2009, data from the Epidemiology of Diabetes and Its Complications (EDIC) showed this to be true even in people who had diabetes for more than 30 years.

Today we have "smart" insulin pumps, rapid-acting insulin, continuous glucose monitors, and even the first step toward a fully automated artificial pancreas. All of these advances serve to keep people with diabetes healthier than ever before.

Our team has been at the forefront of most of these advances in diabetes treatment and control, and we will continue to be there and share all of our knowledge with you as we help you navigate this new path in your life.

Our Team

Our team is made up of the following healthcare professionals:

- *Attending Physicians* – These world-renowned doctors are experts in the field of diabetes and also regularly participate in groundbreaking diabetes-related research trials.
- *Fellows* – Pediatricians who have decided to further their studies and become experts in diabetes and endocrinology.
- *Nurse Practitioners (NP)/Physician Assistants (PA)* – These providers are the core of our team, they provide the bulk of the day-to-day management and see most of the patients in our clinic.
- *Nurses* – Our nurses can be found supporting our providers both during and after your clinic visits.
- *Nutritionists* – Our nutritionists provide expertise in using food to help with the management of diabetes.

- *Social Workers* – Our social workers are available to help with any concerns regarding work, school, coping with the diagnosis, sibling challenges, emotional support and counseling, and anything else that may come up.
- *Research Coordinators* – Our research coordinators support the MDs/NPs/PAs who run the clinical studies that have kept us on the cutting edge of diabetes management.
- *Administrative Support Staff* – Our administrative staff directly support our providers so that they can give the best care possible. These team members are also responsible for answering and triaging calls from families, patients, and other providers.

Our Philosophy

- We believe that diabetes is a condition, not an illness.
- Managing blood glucose levels as close to normal as possible will lead to a long and healthy life.
- We believe that diabetes should NOT get in the way of you doing anything you want to do.
- We believe that successful management of diabetes is possible and our team is here to coach you to success.
- We believe that you will quickly become the expert in your diabetes and will learn to manage this condition as independently as possible.
- We will always be available for consultation.
- We believe that we all have the same goal, to keep you as healthy as possible!

What Is Diabetes?

Diabetes is a condition where the sugar levels in the blood are too high. Sugar, also called glucose, is the body's main source of energy. Without a regular supply of glucose, the body cannot function properly.

Need to Know

Diabetes happens when the body can no longer use sugar for energy.

Type 1 diabetes (T1D) is an autoimmune disorder where the body destroys its own cells that make insulin. You must take insulin (by injection or through a pump) to stay healthy.

Type 2 diabetes (T2D) happens when the body cannot make enough insulin to meet demand – this can be treated with exercise, healthy food choices, pills, and insulin.

The body makes insulin in order to keep blood sugar levels from going up too high. Insulin is a hormone that is made in the beta cells of the pancreas that allows glucose to enter into the body's cells. Diabetes happens when either the body cannot make any insulin or it does not make enough insulin.

There are several kinds of diabetes. The most common types are listed as follows:

Type 1 Diabetes (T1D)

This is an autoimmune disorder. That means that the body's immune system, which usually fights off germs and viruses, attacks and damages or destroys certain cells or organs of the body. In the case of diabetes, the body fights against the beta cells of the pancreas. As the beta cells are damaged the body makes less insulin, and eventually the blood sugars become high when there is not enough insulin around. While people with type 1 diabetes can still make some insulin, especially when they are first diagnosed, they still require insulin therapy to keep their blood sugar in normal range. Some people with type 1 diabetes may ultimately lose their ability to make any insulin.

Right now, we do not know why someone gets diabetes. We know that the ability to develop diabetes can be inherited (passed down from parent to child). However, many people have the same genes, but they do not develop diabetes. We also know that something "triggers" diabetes to happen, but we are not sure what the triggers are.

We do know that diabetes is not caused by eating too many sweets or by something that you or your child did or did not do. Right now, we do not have a cure for diabetes. However, we do have many new ways to manage diabetes so a child can take part in any "normal" childhood activity.

Type 2 Diabetes (T2D)

This is the fastest growing type of diabetes in children. It used to be only found in older people and is associated with being overweight/obese and with not exercising regularly. As we see more and more overweight/obese children, we are seeing more children with type 2 diabetes. Type 2 diabetes usually happens when the extra weight on people keeps their insulin from working the way it should. People with type 2 diabetes need much more insulin than people without diabetes and the pancreas cannot keep up with the extra demand.

Medication-Related Diabetes

Some medications such as steroids or chemotherapy used to treat cancer can make blood sugar levels go very high. When this happens, you need to take insulin to make the sugar levels go back to normal. Many times, once the medication is stopped, the insulin can be stopped too. This can be a temporary kind of diabetes.

Cystic Fibrosis–Related Diabetes

Children with cystic fibrosis (CF) can develop diabetes. While the exact cause is not known, it is thought that chronic inflammation of the pancreas from CF prevents the insulin making cells from working. It is very important that children with CF keep their blood sugar levels close to target levels in order to keep their lungs as healthy as possible.

Need to Know

Glucose is the special type of sugar that the body uses for energy.

All other types of sugar are changed into glucose by the body.

Insulin is a hormone that moves glucose from the bloodstream into the body's cells.

Insulin is made in the beta cells of the pancreas.

The Pancreas, Beta Cells, and Insulin

The first step in managing diabetes is to understand how the body normally handles sugar.

As we explained earlier, sugar is the body's main source of energy. Sugar comes from the food we eat and it comes from the body itself – a steady supply of sugar is made in the liver to be used between meals. The body uses a special type of sugar called glucose. Glucose can be used right away or it can be stored in the liver and muscle cells or changed into fat.

Insulin is made in a specialized part of the pancreas called beta cells. The pancreas is a gland that is found in the abdomen, near the stomach. Besides making insulin, it makes several substances that help to digest and use the food we eat.

At meal-time, the carbohydrate in the food is digested, turned into glucose, and absorbed into the bloodstream. As the sugar levels in the blood increase, the beta cells in the pancreas make more insulin so that the extra sugar can be stored in the liver, muscle, and fat cells. Without this extra insulin, blood sugar levels would go up too high, and the body would not be able to store sugar for later use.

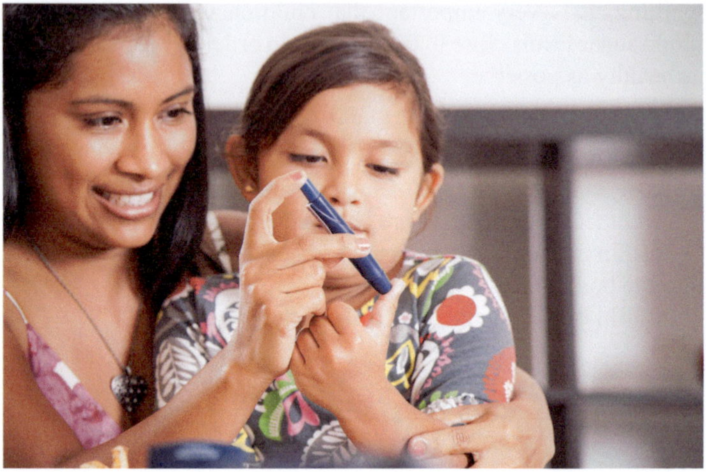

The Ins and Outs of Giving Insulin

All people with type 1 diabetes and many people with type 2 diabetes must take insulin every day in order to stay alive and healthy.

Need to Know

All people with type 1 diabetes must use insulin on a daily basis.

Some people with type 2 diabetes may treat their diabetes with insulin and/or medications and/or exercise and weight loss.

Insulin can only be given as an injection.

People with type 1 diabetes have to take several different types of insulin.

It is extremely important that you know what types of insulin you are on and the ONSET, PEAK, and DURATION of each of these types of insulin.

Insulin can only be given as a shot or with an insulin pump. Insulin cannot be given as a pill because the acid in the stomach would destroy the insulin.

There are many types of insulin available today. All of them can be put into one of four main groups: rapid-acting insulin, intermediate-acting insulin, long-acting insulin, or pre-mixed insulin.

Please note that the insulin plan that you start on initially is not the only way to manage diabetes and we will discuss alternative regimens at future visits.

Rapid-Acting Insulin

This insulin works *right away* to drop the blood sugar.

Brand Names: Humalog®, Novolog® or Apidra®.

ONSET (starts working): 10–15 minutes.

PEAK (strongest effect): 1–2 hours.

DURATION (all used up): 3–4 hours.

Intermediate-Acting Insulin

This insulin works *slowly* to drop the blood sugar.

Brand Names: NPH®, Novolin N® or Humulin N®.

ONSET (starts working): 2–4 hours.

PEAK (strongest effect): 5–6 hours.

DURATION (all used up): 10–12 hours.

Long-Acting Insulin

This insulin is a background or "basal" insulin.

Brand Names: Lantus® or Levemir®, Tresiba®, Toujeo®, Basaglar®.

ONSET (starts working): 2–4 hours.

DURATION (all used up): 14–24 hours.

The nurses here will show you how to administer insulin. Prior to discharge you will need to give your child an injection, so we can be sure you will feel comfortable doing so at home. Historically, insulin was administered by syringe, but now we use insulin pens, which tend to be easier to use.

Using an Insulin Pen

Many families prefer to use insulin pens to deliver doses of insulin. Insulin pens are devices designed to make giving insulin easier. They look much like a pen and cap (this is where the name comes from) and come pre-filled with 300 units of insulin. A knob at the end of the pen "dials up" the insulin dose. In most cases, each click that you hear is equal to 1 unit of insulin. The pens may be reused until they run out of insulin. Most pens are disposable and when you finish the insulin in it (or after it is open for 30 days) the entire pen is thrown out and a new one is started. Some insulin pens are re-usable and are filled with insulin cartridges.

Insulin from a pen is given using a pen needle. This is a small needle that is put on the end of the pen using a twisting motion. The needle can be changed every time that the pen is used, but some patients will use a needle more than once before changing it.

There are many types of insulin pens. You will be given exact instructions on how to use the insulin pen that is prescribed for you or your child. Keep in mind that pens only contain one kind of insulin or a fixed mixture of two types of insulin.

A few points to remember about insulin pens:

- Before every use, it is important to "waste" 2–3 units into the sink or garbage. This is so that you can see that the needle is full of insulin. If this step is not done, the wrong dose of insulin (or no insulin at all) might be given.
- If you do not see drops of insulin come out the needle when you are doing a "waste," repeat the steps until you see insulin come out.
- Count the clicks and look in the dose window to confirm the right dose.
- The pen should be held straight up and down, directly over the place where the injection is going to be given.
- It is important to wait 5–10 seconds after injecting the insulin before pulling out the needle. This allows the entire insulin dose to leave the pen and enter the body.

Need to Know

Insulin is given into the fat tissue.

It is very important to regularly change injection sites.

Intermediate or long-acting insulin must be given at the same time every day, no more than 30-minute difference on a daily basis.

Rapid-acting insulin should be given right before eating.

Injecting Insulin

- Insulin may be given in the arms, abdomen, buttocks, and thighs.
- Insulin is given into the subcutaneous (fat) tissue.
- Remember to "pinch up" some skin and fat.
- Change sites – use a different site for each injection. This helps keep "fat lumps" (AKA lipohypertrophy) from developing at injection sites. The image to the right illustrates options for injection sites.
  - Example: use the arms or abdomen in the morning, and the legs or buttocks at dinner or bedtime.
  - Your provider will check your injection sites at clinic visits to make sure there is no "fat lumps" (hypertrophy) developing.
- Remember to let go of the pinch BEFORE taking the syringe out (otherwise, you may squeeze out the insulin).
- Sometimes people can have an allergic reaction where insulin is injected.
  - You might see redness around the area you gave the insulin.
  - Your child might complain that it itches or that the injection site is red.
  - Redness and itching is most common 3–12 weeks after diagnosis.
  - Call the diabetes team if you have any problems.
  - These reactions usually do not cause bigger problems and often go away after a short time.

- A full body allergic reaction to insulin (body rash, hives, breathing problems) is extremely rare. If you every have any of these symptoms, please call 911 (or your local emergency services) and the diabetes team right away.

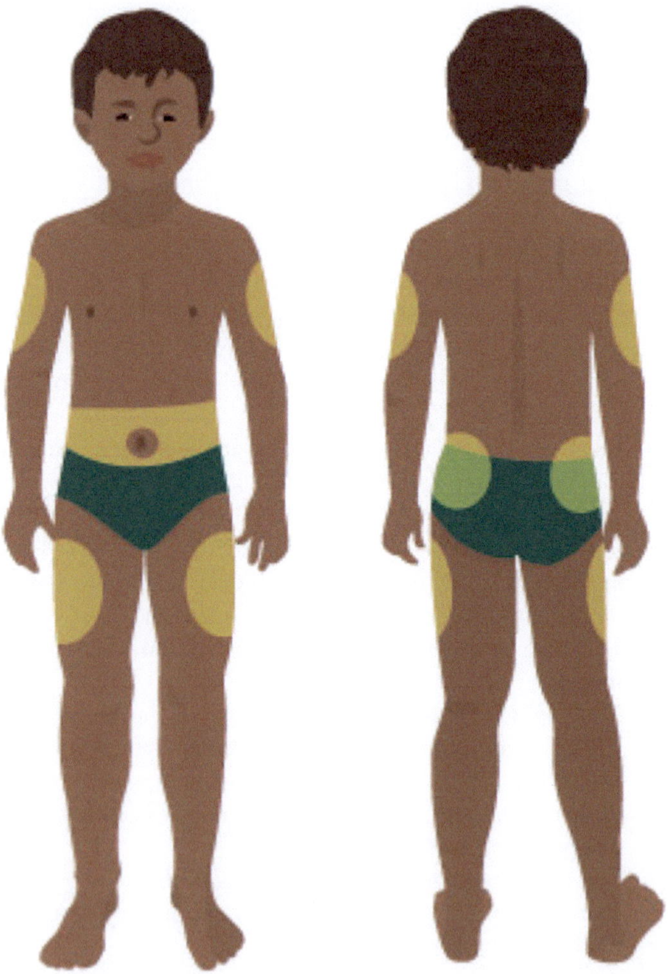

Graphic courtesy of KidsHealth.org.

A Brief Introduction to Insulin Pump Therapy

In brief, insulin pumps are small, computerized devices that mimic the way the human pancreas works by delivering small doses of short-acting insulin continuously (basal rate) along with variable amounts of insulin when a meal is eaten (bolus). Pump therapy can allow greater flexibility in meal timing and in carbohydrates consumed.

Pump therapy was first used in pediatric patients by Dr. William Tamborlane here at Yale in 1979. Therefore, we use lots of pumps in our management of diabetes. Approximately 70–75% of our patients transition to insulin pump therapy. In fact, you likely know someone that wears an insulin pump! Please know that during outpatient visits we will review pump therapy in greater detail and can show you available options, if you are interested. Because we understand that this admission can be overwhelming and involves so many new concepts, we will not go into too many details quite yet.

We do encourage families to reach out to their insurance companies to check on coverage plans and rates. Insulin pumps are typically covered under your Durable Medical Equipment policy.

To see what pumps are currently available, Diabetes Forecast is an online patient-oriented magazine that does a consumer guide each March.

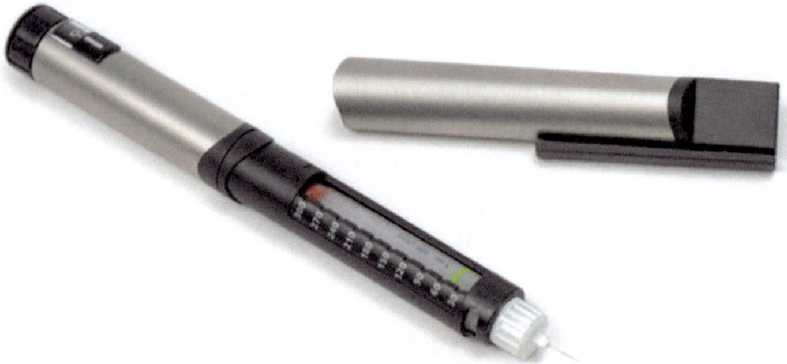

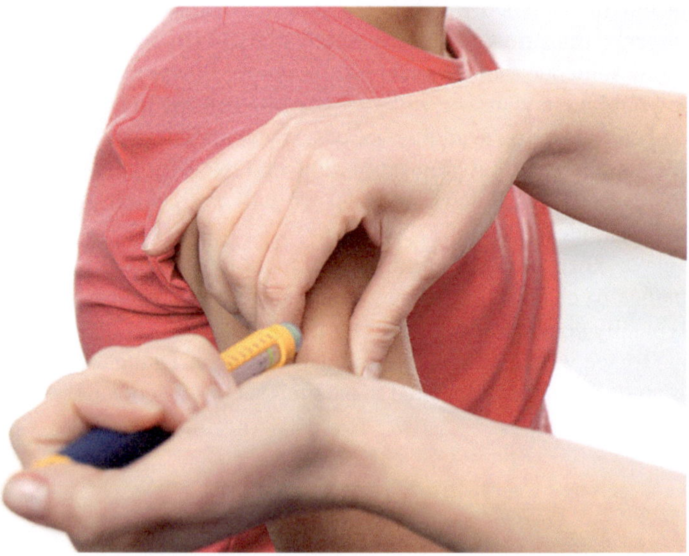

Testing Your Blood Sugar

A very important part of taking care of your diabetes is testing your blood sugar. Knowing your blood sugar level answers many questions such as the following: How much insulin should you take? Is it okay to exercise? Do I need to check for ketones? Should I change my insulin doses?

Need to Know

Blood sugar tests tell us how the insulin is working in your body.

The target range for blood sugar levels is 70–120 mg/dL (unless we have suggested a different range).

The blood sugar level must be tested at least 4 times per day if you are taking insulin.

Extra tests should be done if you do not feel right or you are exercising/being physically active.

Today's blood sugar machines (called meters or glucometers) are very fast and use very small drops of blood. The drops of blood can come from the finger, palms, or sometimes the arm. There are many machines available, and the nurses will help you get started with one.

If you are taking insulin, you MUST test your blood sugar at least four times a day:

- Before breakfast
- Before lunch
- Before dinner
- Before going to bed

You might also need to test your blood sugar at extra times too. These might include the following:

- If you are not feeling right (to check for low or high sugar levels)
- Before exercising
- Before swimming
- In the middle of the night
- If you are having a "sick day"
- If your diabetes team suggests extra testing

How Do I Track My Blood Sugar Levels?

The families who successfully manage diabetes set aside 1 hour every week where they sit together to go over blood sugar numbers and decide whether there are patterns that indicate that a change in the regimen needs to be made. It is a good idea if both parents and the child/teen with diabetes sit down during this time and go over the numbers. It is important for children with diabetes to learn how to look for patterns in their blood sugar levels because someday children with diabetes become adults with diabetes!

Not too long ago, everyone had to write down their blood glucose or blood sugar (BG) numbers because the meters did not have a memory feature. Today's meters can remember hundreds of blood sugar numbers and many meters have computer programs that allow you to download all the blood sugar numbers so that you can study them for patterns in your blood sugar levels.

Right now, at the very beginning, we are going to ask you to write down your blood sugar numbers the "old fashioned" way. This is because we will be speaking with you every day for the first 1–2 weeks, and it is important that you have your blood sugar levels in one place.

Whichever way you choose to look for patterns in your blood sugar, *it is very important that you do it on a regular basis so that you know whether or not your insulin doses are doing their job.*

Sample log book pages may be found in Appendix A at the back of this brochure.

What the Numbers Mean

For people without diabetes, "normal" BG levels" mean that their BG is between a low of 70 to a high of 140–150 mg/dL after eating. For people with diabetes, we try our best to have as many numbers as possible in the "normal" range, but in reality, that is pretty hard to do – in fact, *it is impossible for a person with diabetes to have all of their BG values fall into the normal range.*

What is possible is to have as many BG values in the "normal" range as possible and for the rest of them, we try and keep them as close to the normal range as possible. For children with diabetes, the goal is to spend 60% time there and for adults with diabetes the goal is 70% time there. It is also important to minimize lows (<70 mg/dL). Ideally we like to see this be <3% of all readings.

Another method to describe how well a patient is doing is shown as follows:

Time	Target
Before meals	70–120 mg/dl
2 hours after meals/snacks	<180 mg/dl
Bedtime	90–150 mg/dl

A Brief Introduction to Continuous Glucose Monitors

Sensors, or continuous glucose monitors (CGMs), provide a method to track sensor glucose levels throughout the day and night. A small catheter sits underneath the skin and provides updated sensor glucose values every 5–15 minutes. Some systems real-time and can show the data as it is collected. Others are intermittently scanned and only display data when a user uses their display devices. Sensors are small devices worn by our patients for 7–14 days at a time. They can minimize finger sticks and provide trend information (i.e., is my sensor glucose going up or down). Some systems allow for remote monitoring of data, as sensor data is sent via the cloud and can be viewed in real time by "followers" of the data. This has provided some families with a sense of security, both when the child is at school or even overnight as data is readily available.

We will discuss sensors only briefly during your hospital stay for several reasons. First, it is important that you feel comfortable with diabetes basics. Just like our everyday technology, like our cell phones, sensors can break and we need to assure we can always get glucose data. Additionally, on learning of the diagnosis of diabetes, seeing the data constantly in real time may be overwhelming until you feel more confident about glucose trends and basic diabetes skills. Currently, most insurance companies will only cover the sensor after your second visit (with this hospital admission counting as your first visit). Please note that we typically discuss available technologies in more detail at your first outpatient visit. You can contact your insurance company to see what sensor your plan may cover.

Hemoglobin A1c Levels

To see how your diabetes is controlled, we will measure your Hb A1c level at every clinic visit. This blood test provides an average of your blood glucose levels for the past 3 months. In 1993, results of the Diabetes Control and Complications Trial were published, which showed when HbA1c was as close to normal as possible, there was less risk of developing long-term complications from diabetes.

This is a rough guideline of what average BG each percentile of HbA1c is equal to:

Hemoglobin A1c	Average blood sugar (mg/dL)
6%	120
7%	150
8%	180
9%	210
10%	240
11%	270
12%	300

My Alc at diagnosis

____________________%

Our goal will be to normalize your hemoglobin A1c as much as possible while not having too many low blood sugars. *The pediatric target is to keep HbA1c less than 7.0%.*

Time in Range

In addition to your hemoglobin A1c, time in range helps us better understand your glucose patterns. Time in range is calculated either from data collected on your blood glucose meter or from a sensor (see the section "Testing Your Blood Sugar"). By uploading data from either of these devices, we can determine your time in ranges. There are a number of ways to upload devices, but in our clinic we use Tidepool (See Appendix B for information about Tidepool).

Time in ranges is broken up into a few categories. The categories are as follows:

Time in range	Definition
Time below <54 mg/dL	Level 2 hypoglycemia (very low blood sugars)
Time below <70 mg/dL	Level 1 hypoglycemia (low blood sugar)
Time in range 770–180 mg/dL	In range (at target)
Time above range >180 mg/dL	Level 1 hyperglycemia (high blood sugar)
Time above range >250 mg/dL	Level 2 hyperglycemia (very high blood sugars)

For youth with diabetes, it is recommended to target at least 60% time in target range (this would be ~14.5 hours a day). Importantly, every 5% increase in time in target range is equal to 1 more hour a day at target, which we know is clinically important.

With measures of hemoglobin A1c and time in ranges, we seek to understand how close you are to achieving suggested targets. These measures help us better understand if/how we might want to alter your insulin doses.

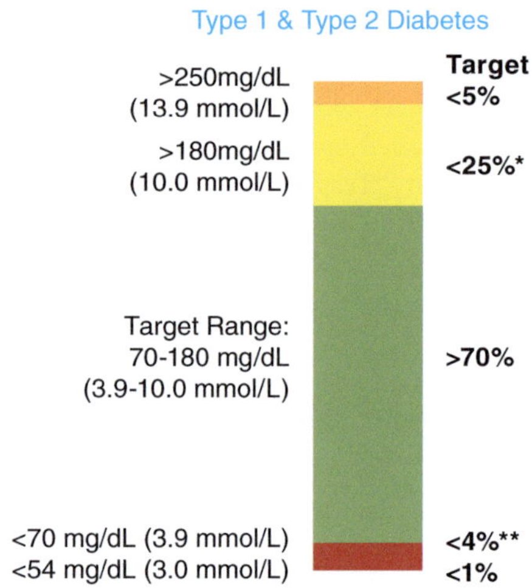

For age <25 years, if the A1C goal is 7.5%, then set TIR target to approximately 60%. (See section "Clinical Applications of Time in Ranges" in the text for additional information regarding target goal setting in pediatric management)
*Includes percentage of values >250 mg/dl (13.9 mmol/L)
**Includes percentage of values <54 mg/dl (3.0 mmol/L)
Figure adapted from Battelino T, Danne T, Bergenstal RM, et al. Clinical Targets for Continuous Glucose Monitoring Data Interpretation: Recommendations from the International Consensus on Time in Range. *Diabetes Care*. 2019;42(8):1593–1603. https://doi.org/10.2337/dci19-0028

New to Know

ANY BG LESS Than 70 mg/dL IS CONSIDERED LOW.

If you can, test first to confirm low BG, then treat.
Treat with FAST-ACTING glucose: 10–15 grams.
WHEN IN DOUBT, go ahead and treat as if the BG is low.

Low Blood Sugar

A low blood sugar is defined as any blood sugar level less than 70 mg/dL, whether or not you have symptoms.

The signs and symptoms can be different in each person, but here are some examples of what you might see or feel when your blood sugar is too low.

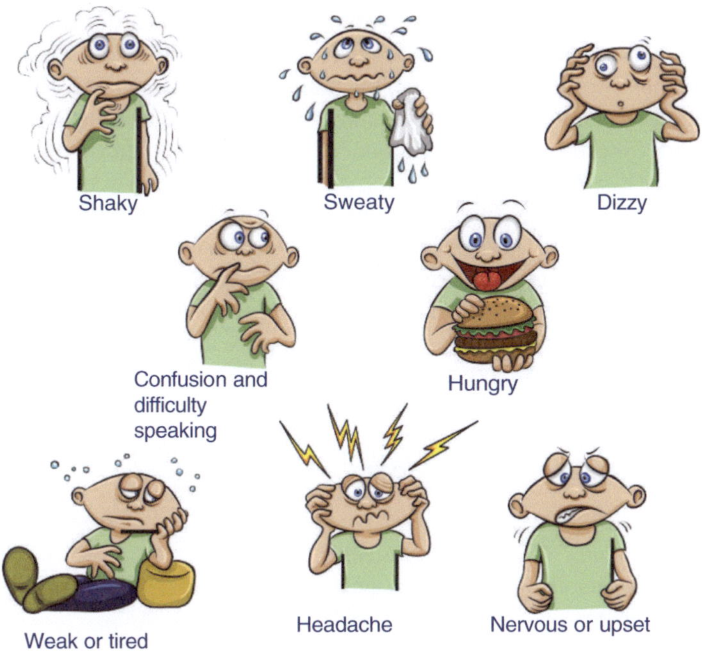
Shaky
Sweaty
Dizzy
Confusion and difficulty speaking
Hungry
Weak or tired
Headache
Nervous or upset

Common causes of low blood sugar:

- Too much insulin
- Too little food
- Too much or unplanned exercise

We cannot prevent all low blood sugar levels from happening, so instead we teach you how to treat the low blood sugar level. In the future, we will teach you how to change your insulin doses if you notice a pattern of low blood sugar levels happening at the same time every day.

Please note that especially during the period initially following diagnosis, it is common to have symptoms of low blood sugars even when the blood glucose is in the normal range. This can occur as blood sugar levels were high prior to diagnosis and the body became used to the higher level. When the blood sugars comes into the normal range, the body falsely warns you that you are low and you can have symptoms. It can take some time for the body to re-set so that symptoms of a low occur when the blood sugar is <70 mg/dL.

If you feel low, but your number is not <70 mg/dL, it is important not to treat with the amount of carbohydrates indicated below. Otherwise, your body will keep alerting you at normal numbers. Sometimes by eating carbohydrate-free foods (protein or vegetables) you can give the body the sense you are doing something but not causing the blood sugar to spike.

Treating Low Blood Sugar

Mild	Moderate	Severe
No symptoms/few symptoms	Symptoms are much stronger	Passed out or having a seizure
10–15 grams fast-acting sugar	15–20 grams fast-acting sugar	
		Glucagon injection
(Choose one)	(Choose one)	Hypokits that needs to be mixed prior to administration
4 oz. (½ cup) juice	4–6 oz. juice	

Mild	Moderate	Severe
4 oz. (½ cup) soda	4–6 oz. soda	Prefilled glucagon pens (gVoke hypo pe)
3 glucose tablets	4–5 glucose tablets	
3–4 Starbursts®	4–5 Starbursts	OR
15 Skittles®	15–20 Skittles	Nasal glucagon (Baqsimi)
1 tablespoon honey	1.5 tablespoon honey	Call 911 or the emergency services in your area
1 tube cake gel	2 tubes cake gel	
½-1 tube glucose gel	1 tube glucose gel	
Fast-acting treatment should be followed by a small snack (10–15 grams) for people on injection therapy if it will be longer than 1 hour until the next meal or snack Suggested snacks: 2 graham cracker squares and 4 oz. milk, 4 peanut butter offer juice and crackers once awake crackers, 1 granola bar, ½ sandwich		Glucagon may cause nausea and vomiting. Once glucagon wears off, the blood sugars may drop low again. In order to prevent this

***A word about severe hypoglycemia:**

Severe hypoglycemia is rare, and it is even rarer when you are newly diagnosed. It is not associated with a specific blood sugar level. Instead, recent research has shown that severe hypoglycemic events most commonly happen after the blood sugar has been low for hours and no treatment has been given during that time. There are times when the risk of having a severe hypoglycemic event is increased and we will work with you to learn how to identify these times and ways to lower the risk.

Need to Know

Review your BG logs to look for patterns over 140–150 mg/dL.

DO NOT PANIC with one very high BG level (>300 mg/dL). One very high level is not an immediate concern as long as you feel OK.

2+ very high levels (at least 2 hours apart) means you need to start figuring out why this is happening and what you can do to lower your BG.

Test for ketones (blood or urine) if you have 2+ very high levels (at least 2 hours apart).

High Blood Sugar

A glucose level over 180 mg/dL is a high level that occurs most often after meals. You do not necessarily need to do anything about this level beyond watching to make sure that a pattern does not develop, where you are above this threshold every day at the same time. Down the road, we will teach you how to make changes in your insulin doses to fix a pattern of high blood glucose levels.

Any level more than 300 mg/dL is considered a very high level. Prior to being diagnosed, you may have regularly had blood sugars over 300. Now, as we begin to check your blood sugar or if you start a sensor, you are bound to see a number over 300 mg/dL at some point. One very high blood sugar level is not a cause for panic; you do not need to go to the hospital for one high blood sugar. Instead, it should serve as an alarm – to let you know you need to do some additional glucose monitoring, maybe check your ketones (see below) and, depending on how you treat your diabetes, it may also mean that you need to take some extra insulin.

Please note that we expect there to be high blood sugars over the coming weeks. This is common as we adjust insulin doses. You will leave the hospital with our "Diabetes Cheat Sheet" which will provide you with a clear plan on how to manage any severe high blood sugars. One of the reasons for our daily phone calls is so that we can adjust your insulin doses if we see trends for high or low levels.

Some people may not notice symptoms of a very high blood sugar level while others will not. These are some common symptoms you might see when your blood sugar level is very high:

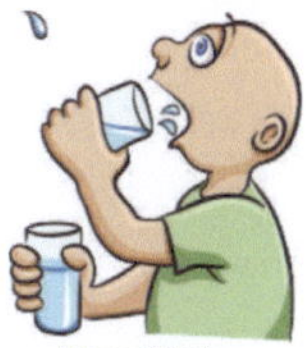
Very thirsty

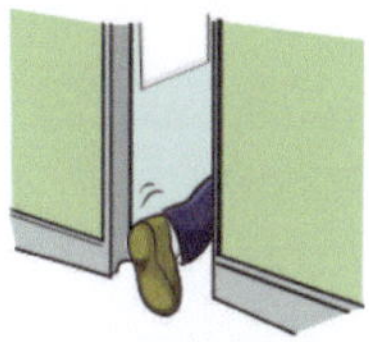
Needing to pass urine more than usual

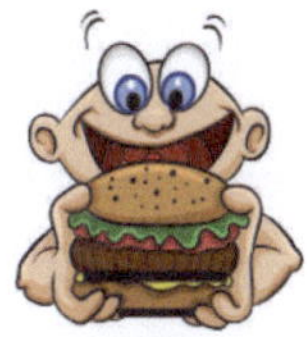
Very hungry

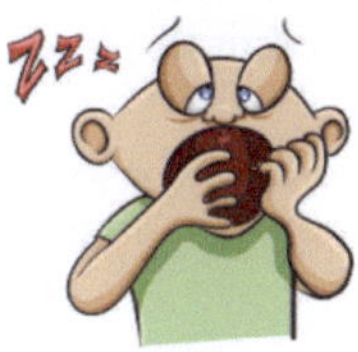
Sleepy

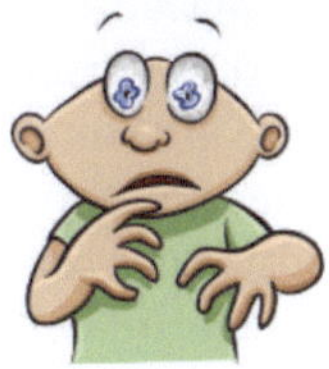
Blurry vision

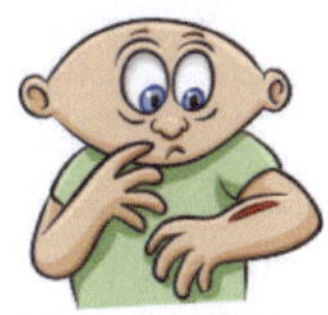
Infections or injuries heal more slowly than usual

Ketones, Ketosis, and Diabetic Ketoacidosis

Very high glucose levels (>300 mg/dL) mean that the body does not have enough insulin around to use sugar as energy. Even though the level of sugar in the blood stream is very high, the body cells may be sending out a signal that they do not have enough energy. In this case, the body will start burning fat to make energy for the cells. This is called ketosis.

Burning body fat for energy makes "leftovers" called ketones. Ketones are a problem because they can build up over several hours and get to such high levels in the body that they make the blood too acidic for organs to work correctly. This leads to a life-threatening diabetes emergency called diabetic ketoacidosis (DKA). Full-blown DKA must be treated in the intensive care unit at a hospital. It is very important to remember that DKA can be prevented.

You must start monitoring for ketones during the following conditions:

- Vomiting (regardless of the blood sugar level)
- 2 blood sugar levels in a row (at least 2 hours apart) that are >300 mg/dL
- "Sick day" – anytime you are too sick to go to school (regardless of your blood sugar level)

There are two methods to check for ketones:
Urine Test: A test strip is placed in urine and taken out. After 15 seconds, you watch for color change and match that to colors on the label to determine the amount of ketones.

Blood Test: Uses a meter and test strip (like testing for your blood glucose level). It provides a number reading that the chart below helps you determine the amount of ketones.

Ketone level	Urine test	Blood test
Normal (negative)	No color change	<0.6
Ketones are minimally elevated above normal	Trace	0.6–0.9
Ketone levels are elevated, serious	Small	1.0–1.5
High levels of ketones, very serious (call diabetes team right away)	Moderate	1.5–3.0
Danger zone (call the diabetes team immediately)	Large	>3.0

Exercise and Diabetes

Physical activity is a great way to lower blood sugar levels. Exercise allows the muscle cells to get sugar from the bloodstream without needing insulin.

People with diabetes who exercise regularly have lower A1c levels and more consistent sugar levels than people who do not exercise. However, for people with type 1 diabetes, no amount of exercise will eliminate the need for daily insulin injections.

Low blood sugar levels can occur during or after exercise, so it is important to know how to exercise safely by carefully managing glucose levels, insulin, and food when being physically active.

Exercise is especially important for people with diabetes and we encourage it, but it must be incorporated into the treatment plan. Please let us know about any physical activities that you might be doing and we will work with you to develop a plan for handling it.

Below are some suggestions about ways to deal with exercise. Remember, everyone's body is different and not all of these suggestions will work for everyone.

Low-intensity activity (i.e., walking, baseball, golf)

- Take your usual insulin doses.
- Test BG before and after exercise.
- If BG <100 mg/dL before exercise: take 15 grams fast-acting glucose (juice or tablets).
- If the activity will last longer than 2 hours, consider having a snack mid-way through of 15 grams carbohydrates.

Moderate-intensity activity (i.e., recreational cycling, recreational swimming)

- Lower that day's insulin dose by 10% (take off at least ½ unit).
- Test BG before and after exercise.
- If BG <150 mg/dL before exercise: take 15 grams fast-acting glucose (juice or tablets).
- If activity is more than 1.5 hours, test BG mid-way through and have a snack of 15 grams of carbohydrates.

High-intensity activity (i.e., competitive swimming, soccer, lacrosse, aerobics, and hockey)

- Lower that day's insulin doses by 20% (take off at least 1 unit).
- Test BG before, mid-way through and after exercise.
- If BG <150 mg/dL before exercise: take 15 grams fast-acting glucose (juice or tablets).

- During activity if BG is between 100 and 150 mg/dL, sip on Gatorade® on breaks. If >150 mg/dL, sip on water.
- Mid-way through have a snack of 15 grams carbohydrates.

Before exercise, if blood sugar is >300 mg/dL, check ketones. If ketones are moderate or large, DO NOT EXERCISE.

What Do I Eat Now? A Basic Guide to Nutrition

The only things we ask you to stay away from are regular juice, regular soda, and regular maple syrup. These three sources of carbohydrates (sugar) make the blood sugar very high but do not have any other nutrients in them.

Need to Know

Carbohydrates are the "sugars" in the food we eat.

Protein and fat do not directly affect blood sugar levels.

"Sugar-free" does not mean carbohydrate free.

"Sugar" is not a bad word.

Stay away from regular juice and soda unless you are treating a low BG level.

All other sources of carbohydrates (starches, sweets, fruits, milk products) are okay. The amount of carbohydrates eaten – not the type of carbohydrates – affects the blood sugar levels the most.

Continue to offer a child with diabetes the same healthy meals you would offer the rest of the family. A child with diabetes does not need special foods or a special diet. You do not need to purchase "diabetic" foods or "low-carb" foods. Sweets are allowed occasionally – just as you would allow for a child without diabetes.

In the beginning, we will ask you to try to keep the amount of carbohydrates in each meal the same from day to day, so we can figure out how much insulin you need. Later on, we will teach you how to adjust your insulin for the amount of carbohydrates that you want to eat.

General guidelines for dealing with food and diabetes

- Eat a well-balanced diet.
- Maintain appropriate weight.
- Try to exercise every day.
- Eat the same amount of carbohydrates every day.
- Eat meals and snacks at the same time every day.
- Do not over treat low blood sugars.
- Adjust insulin according to the food you eat and how much exercise you are doing.
- When exercising, eat snacks to avoid low blood sugars.

Carbohydrate Counting

Carbohydrate is another term for the starches and sugars we eat. Carbohydrates can be found in the following foods:

Bread	Green peas	Punch
Crackers	Potatoes	Regular soda
Grains	Winter squash	Honey
Cereal	Fruit	Syrup
Rice	Yogurt	Molasses
Pasta	Milk	Sugar
Corn	Fruit juice	Candy
Dried beans	Lemonade	

Foods with carbohydrates have a direct effect on blood sugar levels because they are rapidly turned into sugar in your stomach and intestines. Quick-acting sugars such as fruit juice, honey, and regular soda will raise your blood sugar in 15–30 minutes, while slower-acting sugars such as breads, pastas, and beans will take longer, perhaps 30–60 minutes.

Fats, proteins, and other types of nutrients found in foods do not affect blood sugar levels as much as carbohydrates. In fact, fats and proteins can slow down how carbohydrates are absorbed. Children with diabetes should choose a meal plan that is low in saturated fats and has enough protein to promote normal growth and development.

You can find out the number of carbohydrates in any food in one of two ways. You can either use the nutrition facts label found on the back of most packaged foods or you can use a book or look up information online that lists foods and their carbohydrate content.

Using a Nutrition Facts Label to Count Carbohydrates

The information in the nutrition facts label is based on ONE SERVING, but many packages contain more than one serving. Look at the serving size and determine how many servings you are eating. If you eat two servings, you double the number of carbohydrates you are eating. When you are comparing carbohydrates and nutrients between brands, see if the serving size is the same.

The goal of carbohydrate counting is to teach you and your child to measure the amount of sugar in the foods that you are eating. It is very important that the total number of carbohydrates per meal or snack stay the same from day to day. A child does not have to eat the same foods every day as long as the number of carbohydrates stays the same.

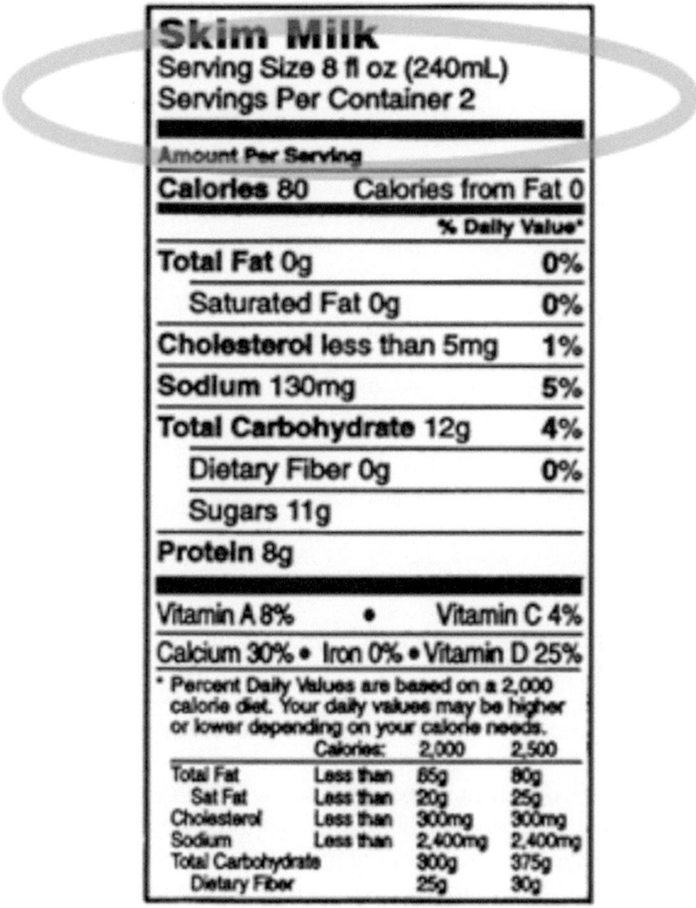
Skim Milk
Serving Size 8 fl oz (240mL)
Servings Per Container 2
Amount Per Serving
Calories 80 Calories from Fat 0
% Daily Value*
Total Fat 0g 0%
Saturated Fat 0g 0%
Cholesterol less than 5mg 1%
Sodium 130mg 5%
Total Carbohydrate 12g 4%
Dietary Fiber 0g 0%
Sugars 11g
Protein 8g
Vitamin A 8% • Vitamin C 4%
Calcium 30% • Iron 0% • Vitamin D 25%
* Percent Daily Values are based on a 2,000 calorie diet. Your daily values may be higher or lower depending on your calorie needs.
Calories: 2,000 2,500
Total Fat Less than 65g 80g
Sat Fat Less than 20g 25g
Cholesterol Less than 300mg 300mg
Sodium Less than 2,400mg 2,400mg
Total Carbohydrate 300g 375g
Dietary Fiber 25g 30g

Suggested Carbohydrate Ranges for Meals and Snacks

Age in years[a]	Total carbs per day	Carbs per meal	Carbs per morning snack	Carbs per afternoon snack	Carbs per evening snack
3–5 years	160–185 grams	30–40 grams	10–20 grams	10–20 grams	10 grams
5–7 years	185–215 grams	45–55 grams	15–25 grams	15–25 grams	<15 grams
7–10 years	215–250 grams	45–60 grams	30 grams	30 grams	<15 grams
10–13 years	250–285 grams	60–75 grams	NONE	30–45 grams	<20 grams
Male >13 years	325–375 grams	75–90 grams	NONE	30–45 grams	<20 grams
Female >13 years	275–300 grams	60–75 grams	NONE	30–45 grams	<20 grams

[a]Children under age 3 should work with a nutritionist on an individual basis

During your stay in the hospital, you will meet with a dietician to review your current eating habits and to create an individualized carbohydrate counting meal plan.

It is normal for you to be hungry right now, and over the next few weeks. Please let us know if you feel you are not getting enough food to eat as we can change your carbohydrate goals so that you are not so hungry. We might need to also increase the insulin doses as well but this is not a problem. Our goal is to match the insulin to what you want to eat instead of making you eat what matches the insulin.

Remember that as you grow you will need more food. That means more carbohydrates too. Every child is different but in general we expect teenagers to need a lot more food than children in elementary school. The table below lists suggested ranges for carbohydrates based on age. This is just a guideline. You will work with the diabetes team to make an individualized plan that works best for you.

Free Foods

There are times when the usual meal plan is not enough and you will be looking for something more to eat. During those times, it is better to reach for foods that do not impact blood sugar levels. For example, as your body gets adjusted to more "normal" blood sugars, you may feel low even though you are note low. That is a great time, to try a free food. Here is a list of foods that may be eaten outside of usual meal or snack times and can help hunger without raising the blood sugar level.

Protein	Raw vegetables	Fats	Sugar-free choices	Other
Beef Chicken Turkey Pork/ham Eggs Cheese Cheese sticks Peanut butter Nut butters Light tuna 1/2 cup nuts	Any type of vegetable is fine Carrots Celery Cucumbers Peppers Broccoli Green beans Lettuce	2–3 tbsp salad dressing 2–3 tbsp dip (ranch or other types)	Popsicles (sugar-free) Hot cocoa (sugar-free) Jell-O® (sugar-free) Crystal Light® (sugar-free)	Dill pickles Olives Broth/ consommé

Sick Day Management

Managing diabetes can be more difficult when a person is sick. Blood sugar levels can run high or low, and the body is under a lot of stress and needs more energy to fight off the germs. When we talk about "sick days," we refer to an illness that is serious enough so that you must stay home from school.

Need to Know

Vomiting is considered a diabetes emergency.

NEVER STOP YOUR INSULIN – call if you think the dose is not right.

During sick days, check your BG and ketone levels every few hours.

If your body cannot get energy from food or sugar, it will quickly start burning body fat and burning body fat for energy leads to the development of ketones. Ketones can build up in the bloodstream and lead to diabetic ketoacidosis (DKA). This is a life-threatening emergency.

Even when you are too sick to eat, you still need insulin. You need enough insulin in your body so you can help prevent the switch from using sugar to using body fat for energy.

Please note that your child can continue to take most medications that they were taking prior to the diagnosis of diabetes including analgesics (Motrin or Tylenol), seasonal allergy medications, etc. If you have any questions about how a new medication might impact sugar levels, please contact our team.

Sick Day Guidelines

- Check the blood sugar every 2–3 hours day and night. *Please review the flowsheets located at the end of this booklet.
- Check ketones every few hours (even if the blood sugar is not high and/or the ketones were negative previously).
- If no vomiting, drink sips of clear fluids:

  - BG <180 mg/dL: use fluids with sugar – apple juice, Gatorade®, ginger ale, regular popsicles
  - BG >180 mg/dL: use fluids without sugar – water, Crystal Lite®, Propel®, diet ginger ale, sugar-free popsicles
- If vomiting is present:
  - Wait at least 1 hour then start fluids very slowly (1 tbsp every 15 minutes for the first hour):

    BG <180 mg/dL: use fluids with sugar – apple juice, Gatorade®, ginger ale, regular popsicles

    BG >180 mg/dL: use fluids without sugar – water, Crystal Lite®, Propel®, diet ginger ale, sugar-free popsicles
- DO NOT STOP INSULIN. You must always take insulin but the amount may change. Call the diabetes team if you need help figuring out how much to take
- If the BG is running very low and you are vomiting or cannot drink anything:
  - Dip your finger into a bowl of table sugar mixed with cinnamon and suck the sugar off the finger.
  - If you have a Glucagon Emergency Kit – draw it up with an insulin syringe.

    Age <2 years old: give 2 "units."

    Age 2–14 years: give 1 "unit" per year of age (for example if age 7 give 7 units).

    15+ years: give 15 units.

    If you have Glucagon Nasal Powder (Baqsimi), you can use it.

Diabetes and School

You spend many hours in school, so it is very important that the school know that you have been diagnosed with diabetes.

Need to Know

Call the school while you are still in the hospital, to let them know about your new diagnosis.

Make sure you have a copy of the Diabetes Medical Management Plan with you when you meet the school nurse.

Make sure your school has enough of your supplies throughout the year.

Put together a "diabetes school kit" – in a plastic box/bin.

Please call our social worker if you have any difficulties getting what you need while at school.

Your teachers, the principal, and school nurse should be told right away. If you ride a bus to school, your bus driver needs to know as well. Sharing this information will help keep you safe and healthy in school and allow you to focus on learning.

Suggestions for School Success

- Call the school while you are still in the hospital and ask to set up a meeting time with the school nurse and/or the principal.
- Make sure you get a copy of "school orders" (called the Diabetes Medical Management Plan) from our team.
  - These orders will instruct the school on how to manage your diabetes while you are there
- Put together a school "diabetes kit" – items you will need to have handy while at school.
  - Extra glucose meter (if you do not have one, just ask us!)
  - Blood glucose test strips and lancet device
  - Juice boxes
  - Glucose tablets
  - Glucose gel
  - Glucagon injection or nasal glucagon
  - Granola bars or other small snacks
  - Ketone strips
  - Bottled water (if you will not drink school water)
- Keep something handy at all times in order to treat a low – younger children usually have juice boxes in the teacher's desk. Older children will carry something in their pocket or their backpack.
- If you are going outside for gym or recess, treatment for a low blood sugar should go with you or with the teacher/aide in charge.

- Make sure to set up a diabetes management plan before you start standardized tests – you should be allowed to test your glucose and take steps to manage your diabetes whenever you need to and you should not be penalized for this.
- Consider discussing a plan with school staff for any lock down drills that might occur. There should be a plan in place in the event that your child cannot leave his/her classroom for an extended period.
- Consider a 504 plan – a legal agreement between you and the school that details how your diabetes will be managed at school.

Mental Health and Diabetes

Diabetes is a task heavy diagnosis, requiring constant mindfulness for those diagnosed as well as their caregivers. Oftentimes, this period can be accompanied by stress and emotional responses can include feelings of being overwhelmed, anxiety, depression, and anger around the condition.

Social Work support is available to all of our patients and their families. In fact, we ask that a social worker meet with all families in the new onset period.

It is completely normal to experience varying emotions, especially during this adjustment period. You may find yourself asking questions such as "Why me?" Our team Social Worker is available to provide counseling related to coping with diabetes. We also consider other impacting factors such as ADHD, existing mental health history, and procedural anxiety. Social work will assist with school planning, work accommodations, changes in the home related to a new diagnosis, and in connecting to community resources. Therapy support is available and encouraged as you navigate this new and challenging life change. Our outpatient team includes specialized social work support, so that even long after the diagnosis you can access these services. Our team is here to support your health, both physically and emotionally.

You can start learning about Diabetes and Mental Health online through:

The Juvenile Diabetes Research Foundation www.jdrf.org/t1d-resources/living-with-t1d/mental-health/

The American Diabetes Association www.diabetes.org/diabetes/mental-health

Leaving the Hospital

Once you leave the hospital, we will continue to support you.

We will continue to speak with you on a daily basis, generally through the first 2 weeks after diagnosis. We ask that you call every day for adjustment of the insulin doses.

Please know that you can also use these calls to ask us any questions that you might have. There is NO SUCH THING AS A DUMB QUESTION! We understand that once you leave the hospital, many questions can come up, so please ask us.

How to Reach the Diabetes Team

Dose adjustment calls

Monday–Friday

- Call 203-785-5831 and press option # 3 to reach our nursing staff.
- Please call between 12 and 2 pm (unless other arrangements have been made).
- Please be prepared to leave a message on our Nurse line and one of our nurses will call you back.
- Please be sure to turn off your caller ID block.

Saturday, Sunday, and Holidays

- Call 203-785-5831 and press option # 1.
- You will be connected to the answering service – please ask them to page the on-call clinician.
- Please call between 12 and 2 pm (unless other arrangements have been made).
- Please have handy all of your BG numbers and insulin doses.
- Please be sure to turn off your caller ID block.

Emergency calls

- A clinician is on call 24/7 to be available for true diabetes emergencies.
- Use this service for the following:
  - Vomiting or extreme nausea
  - Moderate to large Ketones
  - Severe hypoglycemia (treat it first, then call our team)
  - 2+ BG levels in a row over 300 mg/dL, at least 2 hours apart
- In the beginning, if you are not sure if something is an emergency, please call us so we can help you decide – no matter the time, day, or night.
- Call 203-785-5831 and press option #1.
- You will be connected with the answering service – please ask them to page the on-call clinician.
- Please be sure to turn off your caller ID block.

Nurse calls

- Our clinical nurse coordinator is available between visits to answer urgent questions that cannot wait until your next trip to clinic.
- This is a voicemail system and you can expect a call back within 24 hours.
- Call 203-785-5192 to directly reach the voicemail box.
- You may also call 203-785-5831, press option #5 to reach our front desk and ask to be transferred to the voicemail line.

Prescription line

- Please make every effort to ask for prescriptions while you are in your clinic visit.
- If you find you are running out of supplies or need to change your prescription, please use our Nurse's line.
- Please note we will need up to 48 business hours to complete a prescription request.
- Call 203-785-5831 and press option #3 to reach the voicemail box.

All other calls (appointment changes, forms, letters etc.)

- Again we kindly request that you ask for these during your clinic visits but if something comes up before the next visit, our administrative personnel are available to assist you.
- Call 203-785-5831 and press option #5 to reach our main office.

Coming to Clinic

Your first appointment in our clinic is on:

Our location
1 Long Wharf Drive
Pediatric Specialty Center – 2nd floor
New Haven, CT 06511

Please note there is a free parking lot on site. There are spaces in the front lot that are specifically reserved for the Pediatric Specialty Center.

Important phone numbers
Main Clinic number: 203-785-5831
Main Clinic fax number: 203-764-6748

During this first appointment with our clinic, you will meet with one of our nurse practitioners. This first visit is long – sometimes up to 1.5 hours in length. At this and every visit after, we will measure and weigh you, check your blood pressure, and run a hemoglobin A1c test. We will ask for a drop of blood (the same as when you test your blood glucose) in order to run this test.

Please bring your log book, your meter (or meters), and any questions you might have. You may also have the opportunity to meet with our social worker, psychologist, and/or our nutritionist.

The next appointment will be scheduled for 4–6 weeks after your first one. After that, we will see you in clinic every 3 months. Our visits are not "traditional" visits to the doctor. We will only perform a brief physical exam, the bulk of our time together will be spent managing issues related to diabetes. If you have a specific question or concern that you would like to discuss, please let your clinician know at the beginning of the visit.

In our clinic, you have the opportunity to schedule your follow-up appointments either by clinician or by date and time. If you need to come on the same day, at the same time, this can be accommodated. If you prefer to see the same clinician each visit, please let the receptionist know your preference and we will do everything we can to honor that request.

Appendix A

Log Book Pages

Date	Breakfast BG	Lunch BG	Dinner BG	Bed BG	12 AM	3 AM	Other (note time)	Comments

Date	Breakfast BG	Lunch BG	Dinner BG	Bed BG	12 AM	3 AM	Other (note time)	Comments

Date	Breakfast BG	Lunch BG	Dinner BG	Bed BG	12 AM	3 AM	Other (note time)	Comments

Date	Breakfast BG	Lunch BG	Dinner BG	Bed BG	12 AM	3 AM	Other (note time)	Comments

Appendix B

Accessing your Diabetes Data

There are multiple platforms that can allow you and us to view the wealth of data generated from diabetes devices. At Yale Pediatric Diabetes, we use Tidepool to view data needed to make diabetes management decisions. Tidepool is a nonprofit organization that allows for uploading of multiple diabetes devices.

Please hold onto these instructions for future use, we will not need you to upload your data right away as we will be going over blood sugar levels and insulin doses during our regular phone calls. Down the road, this is a very helpful tool and you can refer back to this section to help!

The Tidepool website is www.tidepool.org.

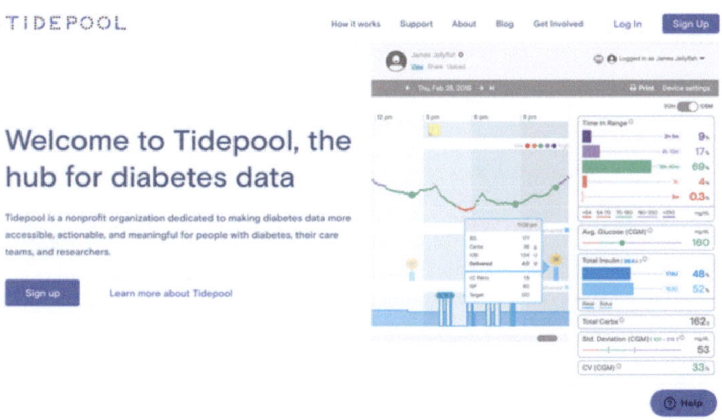

The Yale Children's Diabetes Program
Long Wharf Drive
Clinic office: Pediatric Specialty Center – 2nd floor
Administrative office: Suite 503
New Haven, CT 06511
ynhch.org

Index

W. V. Tamborlane (ed.), *Diabetes in Children and Adolescents*, Contemporary Endocrinology,
https://doi.org/10.1007/978-3-030-64133-7

MIX
Papier aus verantwortungsvollen Quellen
Paper from responsible sources
FSC® C105338
www.fsc.org

If you have any concerns about our products,
you can contact us on
ProductSafety@springernature.com

In case Publisher is established outside the EU,
the EU authorized representative is:
Springer Nature Customer Service Center GmbH
Europaplatz 3, 69115 Heidelberg, Germany

Printed by Libri Plureos GmbH
in Hamburg, Germany